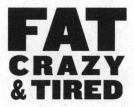

FAT
CRAZY
& TIRED

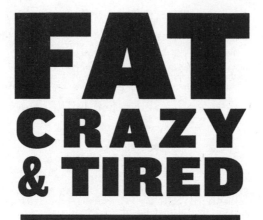

FAT CRAZY & TIRED

Tales from the
Trenches of Transformation

VAN LATHAN JR.

LEGACY
LIT

NEW YORK • BOSTON

Legacy Lit, an imprint of Grand Central Publishing
Hachette Book Group
1290 Avenue of the Americas
New York, NY 10104
LegacyLitBooks.com
Twitter.com/LegacyLitBooks
Instagram.com/LegacyLitBooks

First Edition: April 2022

Grand Central Publishing is a division of Hachette Book Group, Inc. The Grand Central Publishing and Legacy Lit name and logo is a trademark of Hachette Book Group.

The Hachette Speakers Bureau provides a wide range of authors for speaking events. To find out more, go to www.hachettespeakersbureau.com or call (866) 376-6591.

The publisher is not responsible for websites (or their content) that are not owned by the publisher.

Library of Congress Cataloging-in-Publication Data
Names: Lathan, Van, Jr., author.
Title: Fat, crazy, and tired : tales from the trenches of transformation / Van Lathan Jr.
Description: New York : Legacy Lit, 2022. | Summary: "When the Covid-19 pandemic first hit, many Americans coped with the impending crisis the only way they knew how: by stockpiling snacks by the pound and alcoholic beverages by the bulk, and binging Netflix and Hulu until their eyes bugged out. After dedicating years to improving his physical and mental health, media personality and podcast host Van Lathan Jr. soon found himself stuck in a similar boat-surrounded by carbs galore, non-stop exhaustion, and crippling waves of anxiety and depression. A formerly chubby kid who self-identified for much of his life as "the fat friend," Van has struggled with physical and mental health his entire life. He was used to being his besties' wing man on the dating scene, the slack bench-dweller at the gym, and his mother's biggest fan at every meal, especially whenever she served up her infamous mac and cheese with five different kinds of cheese. At 365 lbs, Van hated being fat, but more than anything, he hated himself for being fat. And so, he got to work on healing his anxiety and started shedding the extra weight. Before the pandemic struck, Van had successfully lost 85 pounds-only to gain much of it back during a year that decimated not just his health, but the health of Americans across the country. Fat, Crazy & Tired isn't just about Van's rollercoaster, ultimately unsuccessful journey to an Instagram-able body; it's about the unspoken personal battlefield of attaining and maintaining that good health. Unlike the self-help gurus that push you to go "all or nothing" and "keep it 100," Van argues for us to be happier and healthier at 50% without totally killing ourselves to get there. After all, Van nearly lost his life on what he deems "the Hood Atkins Diet" by indulging on bacon. He also explores the real reasons behind our unending physical and mental health battles-culture, family, and the baggage of life-and demonstrates how we can better understand our bodies by better understanding ourselves. Forget all those self-help books, diets-of-the-week, and extreme exercise fads. "Detox" cleanses? Weight loss pills? Celery juice? No, thank you. Instead, this book provides a close look at how to really take control of your health-in all areas-one step at a time, with patience, compassion, and a dose of humor. If you're DONE with feeling fat, crazy & tired-or you know someone else who is, well then, this book is for YOU"— Provided by publisher.
Identifiers: LCCN 2021053684 | ISBN 9780306923722 (hardcover) | ISBN 9780306923746 (ebook)
Subjects: LCSH: Lathan, Van, Jr.—Health. | Weight loss. | Self-care, Health. | Mind and body. | COVID-19 Pandemic, 2020—Influence.
Classification: LCC RM222.2 .L355 2022 | DDC 613.2/5—dc23/eng/20220107
LC record available at https://lccn.loc.gov/2021053684

ISBNs: 9780306923722 (hardcover), 9780306923746 (ebook)

Printed in the United States of America

LSC-C
Printing 1, 2022

For Van Lathan Sr.

Contents

I

BORN THIS WAY

II
UNLEARN OR BURN

III
HAVING SAID ALL THAT,
I'M STILL FUCKED-UP

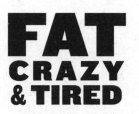

FAT
CRAZY
& TIRED

Are You Fat, Crazy, and Tired, Too?

I f you decided to drop your dollars on this book, let me start out by saying thank you and then follow that up by letting you know that I'm not an expert in anything. I'm not a personal trainer, a psychologist, or a life coach. Every story in this book is simply my experience of getting through the other side of things without losing my shit in the process.

When I moved to LA, I was definitely on the run from EVERYTHING. Hurricane Katrina had just happened, and

I had watched South Louisiana be decimated down to the point that people were wondering where they were going to get their next food and shelter from. It's just a messed-up situation to be in; if you're hungry, you go somewhere and you buy something to cook, but then what happens when there's no food in Walmart? I saw the amount of apathy that it sparked in the rest of the country. We all realized just how quickly things could break down. It pushed me to go out and seek a bigger world, but at the same time, it crystallized for me that I needed to get away from where I was, that there was something that I had to go find. Literally, I told people on a Monday that I was leaving on Thursday, and I left and never lived there again.

A lot of people are able to go through a bunch of different things and still come out on the other side feeling completely okay. I can't do that. It bothers me, it gets to me: I cry, I'll pout, and I'll have a panic attack. I really have to work at it. It took me a long time to even get to a point of working at it. Then I realized that if I wanted to be mentally and spiritually clear, I had to be good with being all of me, with being a cool guy, but also fat, crazy, and tired as fuck.

I care enough about you not to bullshit you about how hard it is to discover who you are, like I have, but know that when you do, there are incredible gems on the other side of being honest with yourself. It wasn't easy to come up with three amazing words for this book title to define myself clearly. Being fat, crazy, and tired has been my healing power. It has gotten me into doing the work every day to be better. When you're willing to work on healing, then you can be an example to those around you to do it themselves.

As we go down this road of healing together, the first thing that I'll say is you're worth every technique, meditation, fad diet, energy drink, exercise, whatever it is, to keep trying. You have to put a value on your healing. Whatever that value is, you're worth that. It's going to cost you money; deep healing can sometimes get in your pockets. It's going to cost you hours out of your day; when you could have been playing video games or having a beer, healing is going to distract from that time. But you're worth it.

There was a time when the paramedics were coming to my apartment in Louisiana so much that they knew me by name. But I learned that the truth of the matter is, it doesn't always have to be that way.

Sometimes people don't want to know the parts of them that aren't perfect. It's a vulnerable thing, and you're afraid you'll be disgusted. It's not a very affirming thing to do if you're doing it right. But the more I get to know about myself, the more I grow, and the more I see how I need to readjust the matrix that is me. The one day I think I have it all figured out, that same day I can think, *Oh my God, I suck.* That's the thing that you start to appreciate when you really start to know yourself, when you really start to get into who you are.

Now that I have sprung from the prison of why I'm supposed to hate being fat, crazy, and tired and fight for perfection, I've written this book to tell everyone else how to blow the joint. And I don't really give a fuck how we have to do it, either. If we have to tunnel out, we're getting out. If we have to behave perfectly for the parole board, we're getting out. If we have to write letters to the judge every day to get a pardon, we're getting out. The world isn't tolerating us because we're fat and crazy. The world needs us! We live in a huge, interconnected community of people, where everyone has something to offer. Let's get free, y'all.

I

BORN THIS WAY

The Wally World Nightmare

In 2004, my father would not stop peeing. There were rivers and rivers of urine flowing from him. As I watched him, I began reflecting on the marvels of the human body. I thought about Mary Lou Retton's body contorting through the air during the 1984 Summer Olympics, Vince Carter's reverse 360-degree windmill in the 2000 dunk contest, and David Blaine encasing himself in a block of ice in New York City for more than sixty-three hours that same year. As amazing as all of those feats were, they were easily getting lapped by my father's bladder.

It would start with a liquid thud as the urine assaulted the plastic container. Then it would sonically evolve to a gurgle as the container filled to capacity. After that, there was the sudsy sound as he topped off at the end. This went on for hours. He just wouldn't stop pissing. I was scared. It wasn't the peeing that was scaring me. What was scaring me is that my father was in a hospital bed.

I'd gotten a call from my sister earlier that day that he'd been struggling. His heart rate was high, his breathing was labored, and his ankles were so swollen that his shoes wouldn't fit on his feet. When I arrived at the hospital and made my way to his room, I barely recognized him. Dad had been my superhero all my life, and like most superheroes, he had a uniform. He wore a cowboy hat on his head, a gigantic western buckle on his belt, and attached to that belt, the ultimate don't-fuck-with-me symbol: a .357 Magnum revolver. Add a pair of ostrich-skin boots to his feet, and that was my dad, all day, every day.

But that wasn't him in that hospital bed. From the top of his head, I could see the gray hair coming in. His feet were bare. Next to the bed were my size 15 Nike flip-flops, the only thing he could fit his feet in to get to the hospital. His uniform was gone, and so was the confidence that came with it. His eyes were normally resolute, representing the resolve of a man who had an answer for every question. Living with someone who's never wrong is generally annoying as fuck, especially when that person isn't humble about it. If they were an asshole, you could hate them for being right. But Dad was humble, and that's much harder to deal with when you're wrong.

The confidence in my father's eyes was totally gone. It was replaced with something I'd never seen in them before: fear. He had no faith that the next breath was going to be there when he drew it.

My father had congestive heart failure. The piss Olympics were taking place because his heart was failing to properly move nutrients in his body, which had led to the fluid buildup. Whenever my dad would go into heart failure, the marathon pissing would come about. This time, he eventually stabilized, but then came the cavalcade of doctors. There was one doctor to explain CHF to him and another one to talk about his treatment options. Then there was the doctor that I called the Health Fairy.

I called this guy the Health Fairy because up to that point in my life I'd never met someone so excited about eating right. It was annoying as fuck. He'd talk about cauliflower like it was fried catfish. He was gushing about pumpkin seeds like they were Popeyes chicken. He was talking about a weird invention called kale.

At this point, it was me, my dad, and my sister in the room. He was speaking a different language. He was talking about health in a way that made it seem like my dad was fighting a battle with every meal he put in his mouth.

It was obvious the Health Fairy took his own advice. This fucker was LEAN. Not like a regular-dude comfortable-with-his-shirt-off-at-the-beach lean, either. This guy was like offensively lean. Like Will Smith in *I Am Legend*. You know that little V pelvis thing? Some regular people have that, which is depressing enough for the rest of us. But some people actually have visible veins in the V thingy. That's when the rage comes in. That's when you start to think, *Why do I have to be shirtless in the same universe as that person?* This was the Health Fairy. He was lean, and it was bothering us. Still, we were afraid enough to listen to his spiel intently. He eventually finished, referred us to a few health websites, and then he left. My father then tilted his head to the side, looked at me, and said, "Damn. I ain't know all that."

He didn't know he was killing himself. I didn't, either. As I sat there watching this, I was obese myself, weighing in at around 365 pounds. I'd very soon find out that my blood pressure was dangerously elevated, making my father's current condition basically a prediction of the future outcome for me. We were both machines careening down a road to a total health disaster—only his car had a twenty-five-year head start. My father didn't want to kill himself. He didn't want to be endlessly pissing in a bedpan and gasping for air. But this is something he'd totally done to himself, and I was following suit. Do you know what it means if you do something without knowing you're doing it, every day, without fail? It means the outcome from what you're doing isn't your fault, even though you're responsible.

IT'S NOT YOUR FAULT.

For a lot of people, this conclusion is hard to believe. Some people may see us actively making poor health decisions, and say, "Hey! That's the reason these people are fat!" It seems obvious to them that if we eat terribly and hardly work out, we'll find ourselves on the higher side of the scale. If we didn't want to be fat, we should eat better. It's that simple, right? HELL THE FUCK NO!

Our society is obsessed with looking good. In order for Zac Efron or Jennifer Lopez to be who they are, there must be people like me for society to compare them to. If I don't have a little extra around my belly, they don't get to look amazing. And it's fucked-up how factors beyond a person's control can lead them to spending life in a body-image prison and despair.

It's really weird for anyone to compare themselves to a Hollywood star in the looks department. It would be like a rec-league basketball player getting pissed off that he's not Kobe Bryant. News flash: Kobe didn't play basketball after his evening shift at work. KOBE WAS BASKETBALL. Some big-name celebrities legit have people who draw their blood and develop diets around their insulin barrier. But we judge ourselves that we're too weak to put down the package of Twinkies and do some push-ups. The blame that the rest of society puts on regular people with extra fat turns to SHAME for us all.

Shame is the number one driving force behind a seemingly never-ending cycle of bad decisions. For me, food is the way that I cope. The worse I feel about myself, the more coping I need. More coping, more weight, and more weight, more coping. Before I know it, my feet are invisible. We all grew up with situations that created who we are. We've all been judged for becoming exactly who those circumstances led us to be. We then let them define us. We believe the bullshit everyone else says about us. We then make all of that who we are.

For those of you who are flogging yourself because of the body you're in, I have a reprieve for you: It's not entirely your fault. Your diet—your eating habits and your relationship with food—was most likely given to you. You received it first from your parents and then from the culture of the community you grew up in. And your parents' idea of a diet was probably heavily influenced by the culture they grew up in. This is a *Chicken or egg first?* theory. I'm sure by the time you had control over your diet, you were likely an adult. Forming healthy habits has less to do with learning something and more to do with UNLEARNING it.

I call this phenomenon *Good Will Hunting* disease, after the 1997 Academy Award–winning movie starring Matt Damon, Ben Affleck, and the late Robin Williams. While I will be offended if you haven't seen it, I'll still begrudgingly do a quick recap. Matt Damon plays Will Hunting, a slightly sociopathic math genius with great hair. Ben Affleck, in his finest pre–*The Town* performance, plays Matt's ride-or-die buddy, Chuckie. Everyone in Will's crew knows he's basically Stephen Hawking. But rather than encourage him to do something crazy like, I don't know, GO TO SCHOOL, they maraud around with him, get wasted, and beat the shit out of guys they went to elementary school with. Matt Damon is charming as fuck in this role. But make no mistake—Will is a criminal.

There's a scene in the first half of the movie where, after Will is arrested for assaulting a police officer, he stands before a judge and tries to get out of the charge. During that scene, we learn that this is not Will's first time before a judge. He had been arrested for a litany of charges throughout his teens and early twenties. After Will does a Mike

Tyson on a police officer, the judge decides Will has to go to jail. However, Will is rescued from a stint in state prison because he solved a superhard equation on a whiteboard at MIT, where he worked as a janitor. When the professors realize it was Will who solved the problem, they pull some strings to get him released, on the condition that he work with them to solve advanced math. There's one catch, though: Will has to see a therapist. If he doesn't see a therapist, the deal is off.

Up to this point in the movie, you've seen Will's behavior, and you pretty much take for granted that he's a total fuckup. He's violent, irresponsible, and shiftless. If not for the fact that he's likely the smartest man alive, NO ONE would want to be Will Hunting. It's through the relationship with the therapist, played masterfully by Robin Williams, that we learn something. We learn that given what Will has been through, this version of Will Hunting is the BEST possible version of him. We learn about the savage abuse Will endured as a child. We understand why Will is so fiercely loyal to his crew of South Boston hell-raisers and why he's down to scrap for them at the drop of a hat.

As the movie progresses, we learn more about his past experiences. The more we discover about Will, the more we now can't understand how he could NOT be fucked-up. The climactic scene in the movie is when Will has a teary-eyed breakthrough. If you watch this scene and do not cry, you are legitimately a demon soul. A wall of emotion breaks down as Will Hunting finally stops blaming himself for the past that was created for him. It's powerful because Will doesn't want to do it. He wants to believe he's the problem. He wants to believe he's broken. He believes that he's flawed and fucked-up. Those characteristics are part of not only who he thinks he is, but who the world thinks he is as well. He can't let go of the old him until he accepts the fact that it isn't his fault. I mean, the guy was a genius, but he couldn't get out of his own way until he realized that there was a perfectly good reason he wasn't where he wanted to be in life. And up to that point, the reasons were bigger than him.

When I was walking around at nearly 370 pounds, I wasn't aware of my weight. You might be wondering, *How in the world is that possible?* But it's easier than you think when you're from Baton Rouge. Baton Rouge is my hometown, and I love it to pieces. It's too small to be a big city and too big to be a small town. Baton Rouge is a place where real people live. There ain't no fake smiles or manufactured hospitality. That's partly because unlike our jazzier neighbor to the south, New Orleans, we don't *need* anyone to visit. In fact, we are often annoyed by outsiders.

There's one thing Baton Rouge has in common with the rest of the state, though, and that's a very specific relationship with food. In 2021, according to a study conducted by financial website WalletHub, Baton Rouge was the third-fattest city in America. That's actually an improvement, because in 2015 we won it all. A Gallup report released that year ranked us the fattest city in America, with a shocking and sad 36 percent of Baton Rouge residents being deemed obese.

Why my home state is so overweight is complicated. You might think the reason we're so bloated in Baton Rouge is because of our world-famous Louisiana cuisine. You've heard about the gumbo, jambalaya, crawfish étouffée, beignets, red beans and rice, hog cracklings, and king cake. Well, I'm here to tell you there's even more food you DON'T hear about, including boudin, boudin balls, muffulettas, hog's head cheese, pecan candy, and andouille sausage. These foods are all staples as well, and we love them. Add these favorites to our fried po'boys, and how could we not be a little fluffy? It would seem to make sense that a great food culture equals fat people, right? Except for the fact that Louisiana isn't the only place on the globe with world-famous and not-so-light cuisine.

Italy, for example, is the home of pasta, pizza, wine, and sausage. (Bologna is named after a city in Italy, which I bet that city wishes it could change!) So they have to be portly, too, right? Except they're not. Italians are among the slimmest people in Europe. Italy's obesity rate is less than 20 percent, along with Switzerland's, according to the most recent statistics from the CIA, while the French—Louisiana's distant ancestral cousins, whose diet seemingly consists of bread, cheese, and wine—have an obesity rate of less than 22 percent, which is much lower than the obesity rate for the United States overall: 36 percent. These European countries are famous for indulging, so why can they fit into the trendy clothes in Zara, and Louisiana can't? That's because you have to look at culture in a holistic picture, and food is only one part of it.

Culture is about not just what you eat, but how you eat, when you eat, and what it means to eat. One aspect of the culture in Louisiana, and in the South in general, is poverty. Poverty shifts the dynamic for obesity in staggering and saddening ways. Your diet becomes reactive to your pockets, and not proactive to your health. Poor people also tend to work longer hours for less pay. When the head of a household chooses Church's Chicken to feed the family with a twelve-piece meal for $12.99, this isn't just the cheapest option. For many poor and underemployed people, it's the only option. This is important to realize, because it speaks to something imperative to having a healthy diet: choice.

In order to become a health-conscious person, you must have the ability to weaponize your choice. It's got to be a thermonuclear device that destroys every single bad eating or exercise habit you've ever formed. Now, we'd all like to imagine that we have the full gamut of choices available to us at any given time, but that's not true. The reality is we're human, and we tend to make choices based upon ease of access. If you live in an apartment complex that has a Whole Foods, you're probably going to stop in once in a while for some organically sourced salmon steaks. If you live next to a Popeyes, you're probably going to try their uberpopular chicken sandwich.

While either person could venture outside of their neighborhood to make better choices, there's this little thing called life that sometimes gets in the way. The choices I grew up with in Baton Rouge were decidedly less healthy than the ones I have now. When you add in the relative poverty of my early family life, there wasn't just a chance I'd be obese—I was actually predisposed to it.

I remember the day I first realized I was obese. It's one of the most crystal-clear memories I have of my life. Do I recall the day I lost my virginity? Nope, can't tell you much about it. Can I tell you about my first day on national television? Nah, don't remember that day, either. But I remember, with startling accuracy, the day I first began to wear the shame of being an obese man in America. And it happened at Walmart.

It was an early morning, I'd just gotten home from working at Best Buy, and I hadn't made it out of the car just yet. I had a fresh bag of McDonald's with me, and I was looking forward to crushing it when I got inside my house.

As I was getting out of my 1993 Ford Taurus to make my way inside, I felt something in my chest. My heart was pounding, and I was also slightly out of breath. I stood there for a second in the crisp Louisiana morning air, almost laughing at myself. It was actually sort of funny that I was winded from getting out of the car; I was allowing myself to have some fun with it. But once the smile drained from my face, I had a question in my mind that had gone unanswered for years. I know now that this unanswered question contributed to both my waistline and my overall blindness about my health. The unanswered question was: How much do I weigh?

In order to answer this question, I knew I'd have to travel to where the scales were, and that would take me to Walmart. I decided not to wait another minute. I turned around on my porch, got right back into the car, and took my big ass over to Wally World.

My first motivation for that trip was knowing right then and there the number on the scale that I had been avoiding, or else I could possibly never have the courage again. Before becoming obese, I'd been an athlete all my life, and facing the reality that I couldn't even get out of the car without breaking a sweat was now really messing with my mind. I also figured that since it was ten o'clock on a weekday, Walmart would be pretty empty, which meant no one would see the fat dude standing on the scale.

When I arrived at the store, it *was* empty. After a little searching, I made my way to the aisle with the scales. My broke-ass twenty-three-year-old self wasn't going to buy a new scale, but there was no way in hell I was going to stand on a scale in full view of anyone who happened to walk by. I decided the best way to get some alone time with a scale was to take it to a place no one would bother us—the bathroom.

I grabbed the first scale I saw, and I started toward the men's room. I almost made it, but it wasn't meant to be. Just as I put my hands on that germ-filled door, I heard a deep voice yell out, "SIR, YOU CAN'T TAKE MERCHANDISE IN THERE."

I turned around and saw a Walmart employee. And not just any Walmart employee—one of THOSE Walmart employees. You know, the type that takes any infraction of store policy as a threat to freedom everywhere. Granted, I have to admit that it was a weird scene. Here I am, a huge Black man in a Best Buy uniform taking a scale into the bathroom. You certainly don't see that every day, and this stalwart protector of retail integrity wasn't having it.

I replied, "I just want to weigh myself. Is that cool?"

I put on my best Kool-Aid smile here, and it had absolutely zero effect on him. He looked at me with a face full of snarling rage and said, "No, you cannot take the merchandise into the bathroom."

I was now facing my big nightmare, but I had gone too far to turn back now. I put the scale on the ground, took my keys out of my pockets, and boldly started to step on. When Walmart guy saw that I wasn't going to be deterred, he barked at me, "Well, if you're gonna weigh yourself anyway, take your shoes off."

"Why?" I asked.

"Your shoes weigh a lot. If you want an accurate number, you should take 'em off. You should really take off all your clothes."

I took a minute with that last statement. I was trying to decide why a store employee had asked me to disrobe. I concluded that it was because he was a know-it-all type, and not because he wanted to see some skin.

I finally decided to take off my shoes and step on the scale. When I looked down, the number displayed was 50. I remember relief washing over me. I obviously weighed more than fifty pounds, but that low number made me feel I was closer to a lower weight than a higher one.

I looked at Walmart man and said, "Shit, it's broke. It says I weigh only fifty pounds."

I'll never forget the look on his face. He was sad. He knew he had to tell me something that was going to be difficult for me to hear. I could tell because his entire disposition changed. He'd been loud and admonishing when he talked to me about the scale before, but he was totally different now. He walked close enough to me where no one would hear him and said, "This is a three-hundred-pound scale. Anything after three hundred, you add the new number on. If the scale reads fifty pounds, you weigh three-fifty."

It's difficult to write what my next thoughts were, because I don't have the words to accurately describe the shame, disgust, and panic I felt. Walmart dude saw my shame, though.

He looked at me and said, "Listen, these scales aren't calibrated. You normally do that when you get them home. It's very possible it's not right. It could be up to forty pounds off."

I didn't reply to him. I didn't pick up the scale. I just walked out of the store. When I got back to the car, my now-cold McDonald's breakfast was still there. The smell held my car hostage. Food was the only thing that was always there for me when I needed it. In that moment, that sausage biscuit with cheese was right on time. I downed it and felt immediately better. However, I couldn't help but think about what Walmart guy had said. Could the scale be off?

Was I really 300, 310, or maybe even 320 pounds? I was sure I couldn't be almost 400 pounds. But I had to know.

Back into the fray I went; this time, I'd go to a different place that I knew would have a more accurate scale. I drove to GNC. At that time, GNC had huge digital scales in the front of their stores that you could use for a quarter. I used those scales to track my weight when I was playing ball in high school. They were more accurate than the scales we had in the locker room. I didn't initially go to GNC this day because immediately after using their scales, without fail, there would always be a kinesiology major with 10 percent body fat trying to sell me supplements. That type of soul-eviscerating scenario is precisely what I'd wanted to avoid. Since nothing could be more embarrassing than the scolding and then pity from the Walmart guy, I basically said, "Fuck it!" and headed to GNC.

When I got there, I located the 10-percent-body-fat sales associate behind the counter. He was lean as hell, and he had some acne on his neck that suggested he was into some other things than what GNC had on its shelves. I asked him if the scale was accurate, and he responded, "Hell yeah. Weighed myself this morning, and I'm two-twelve, solid."

After thinking about how I hadn't asked him how much he fucking weighed, I stepped on the scale. I closed my eyes while the numbers went up, instead of choosing to look at the verdict in one fell swoop. It turns out the Walmart warrior was right. The scale at Walmart *was* wrong. It was light. The GNC scale showed 367 pounds. There was no running from it now. It was a reality. I stepped off the scale, walked back to the car, opened the door, got inside, and cried.

2

Grits, Grease, and Goodness

Perhaps the best example of how growing up in Baton Rouge affected my weight is a local convenience store called Rainbow Express. (In full disclosure, I'm having a slight writing crisis right now. I have to describe Rainbow Express, a place I absolutely loved, but it's impossible to do so without extraordinary shade.)

Rainbow Express was a small, dirtyish convenience store on Gardere Lane, where you could get fake FUBU jerseys, stale chips, and the most glorious po'boys the Lord hath made. Other than the outstanding taste of the po'boys, everything about Rainbow Express was a mystery. They had brands you hadn't seen in years. I'm pretty sure if Rainbow Express were still around right now, you could walk in there and get a can of Tab soda or a New Coke. We never knew how they found these long-defunct and rare products.

But the biggest mystery of Rainbow Express by far was the family who owned it. It took the entire neighborhood years to realize the owners lived on-site in rooms behind the main establishment. Despite their living in the community for years, we NEVER saw the owners or their family members outside of the store. This included their school-age kids, who we never saw at any of the local schools. It felt like everyone who worked at Rainbow Express magically materialized when you walked into the store and then ceased to exist as soon as you left.

One of the first things I noticed in LA was that every place that serves food has to have a letter grade from the health department prominently displayed in the window. An A-rated restaurant means the place is clean, sanitary, and has no vermin infestation. A B-rated restaurant means the place has some issues that need to be cleaned up but it is mostly okay. I've never actually seen a C-rated restaurant in my life. No one I know even eats at the B-rated places, making the financial survival of a regularly C-rated place a fantasy not even Stephen King could cook up.

I don't want to speculate what Rainbow Express would have been rated if these letter grades had existed when I was growing up. But it's important to state that it wouldn't matter at all, even now. The po'boys at Rainbow Express were so singularly fantastic that I'd eat them even if they came with a 25 percent risk of the flu.

What made the Rainbow Express po'boy so good is the same thing that makes a lot of the food I love from home so good. It's sublimely low-quality. It doesn't boast fresh wild-caught catfish or shrimp. It's not on a garlic-glazed gluten-free piece of French bread with a mayonnaise aioli. It's pure neighborhood food. It's affordable and delectable fare, consumed by businesspeople and crackheads alike. The entire neighborhood is proud of it and will go to physical battle with anyone who claims their spot is better.

For me, Rainbow Express wasn't a choice—it was part of my diet. It was a place that no matter how many times you ate there, there was a sense of comfort and joy in the fact that it would never let you down. Also, the po'boys at

Rainbow Express were only five dollars. They were so big that it would hold you down the entire day if you ate it one half at a time.

So here you have food that is cheap and good, and eliminates your hunger. At that point, the sandwich becomes more than food. It becomes a societal elixir for an economically depressed area.

But, in addition to Rainbow Express, there were also the $1.99 fried turkey legs from the Cajun Mart, the $3.99 double bacon cheeseburger meal from Fast Track, and, of course, the plethora of affordable delights from the deli section of the Piggly Wiggly. When I was formulating my ideas about food, these readily available, fast, and cheap choices, along with the AMAZING food my mother made (which we'll get to very soon) is what I based my ideas on. At that time, I only thought about what was cheap, tasted good, and made me as full as I could possibly get. I call this portion-'n'-price syndrome—PP syndrome, for short.

Normally, the cheaper food is, the more we want of it. Inexpensive establishments in places like Baton Rouge can give you more because it's cheaper for them to buy their ingredients. The more economically depressed you are, the more you need out of every meal. I didn't realize I was obese because where I grew up so many people were also overweight.

What does all this data tell you? It tells you that when I was born to Chrystal Ellis, a modern dancer, and Van Terry Lathan Sr., an ex–college baseball player, I was already facing an uphill battle against fat. I was born into a culture of obesity and a place where food is a religion. The unique mix of French, Spanish, West African, Amerindian, Haitian, German, and Italian influences in my state had given birth to a gorgeous and deadly caloric temptress called Cajun cuisine.

In Baton Rouge, we're proud to eat, proud to feed visitors, and desperate for those visitors to tell everyone how no other place on planet Earth comes close to what we can do with flavor. We use food for celebration, for consoling each other, and, believe it or not, for currency.

I got this lesson early on in a place where a young Black kid growing up in South Louisiana learns many of his social lessons: at a funeral. When I was about six years old, my great-great-grandfather—the man who raised my father—passed away. He was a giant in our family, and his homegoing was a can't-miss event. His homegoing service took place where my dad grew up, across the Mississippi River in a tiny town called Maringouin. More than 86 percent of the residents who live in Maringouin are Black, and there's a reason why. In 1838, the Jesuit order of the Catholic Church sold around 272 enslaved people they "owned" in Maryland to southern buyers in Louisiana. Their goal was to generate cash for a struggling institution called Georgetown University. Many of the descendants of those slaves live in what is now Maringouin.

It was at Big Papa's posthomegoing feast that I first realized how important food was to my family. I was looking around at relatives I'd never seen before and being introduced to people telling me how big I'd gotten. Then, suddenly, I heard something. The memory is hazy, but I do remember a female voice saying something like, "I can't believe she brought that dry-ass jambalaya up in here."

Now, while a lot of the players in this scene have since joined Big Papa in the sweet by-and-by, some of them have not. In order to avoid a bloody family civil war, the aunt in question will not be named in this book. What will be mentioned is what happened next, which was incredibly predictable. I found my father, surrounded by male cousins and uncles, and said loudly and proudly, "Auntie got some dry-ass jambalaya."

I've never taken down a room faster. Hats fell off of

heads, beer spilled on the ground, and the I-can't-breathe laughter around me was almost frightening. These guys were stuttering, rolling, grabbing each other, and flailing everywhere. I was superconfused.

I wasn't trying to joke about anything. I was doing what kids do, which is to repeat every inappropriate and hurtful thing they hear, with zero remorse. I can't remember who among my family was laughing the hardest. Could've been my uncle Jimmy. Maybe it was my uncle Craig. Perhaps it was Cousin Snook. But what I do remember is there was one person noticeably NOT laughing, and that was my father.

Precocious as I was, I didn't have the words at that point for the look on his face. But luckily for you, now I do. The look was pure horror. His eyes were wide and shifting from side to side. His brow looked panicked and tense. My dad hates clowns, and the look on his face was as if he'd lifted my mother's veil on their wedding day and saw Pennywise from *It*. He grabbed me, picked me up by my arm (it was a different time—relax), and manifested a quiet spot in a room of two-hundred-some Lathans.

He looked at me, very intently, and said, "Son, your uncles are fucking clowns, you hear me? Don't ever laugh at your auntie's cooking. Ever. It would hurt her so much if she knew you said that. You don't want to hurt her, right? She works hard, and she does her best. If it ain't like your mama's or your grandmama's cooking, then that's okay. She puts love into everything she makes. If you tell her that her food doesn't taste good, it's like telling her you don't love her."

Later in life, I realized two things about this moment. One, this auntie was by far my dad's favorite sister and he'd taken it personally that I'd insulted her cooking. Two, the laughter from the cousins and uncles wasn't just from my comedy. They'd been waiting for someone to say it. The laugh was the release of a family secret, and that secret had to do with jambalaya that no one really wanted to eat but ate anyway.

The lesson my father taught me that day is that food is an emotional extension of people. It was them telling and showing you that they love you. We were saying goodbye to a man who'd built our family, and my aunt was telling everyone how much she loved them with her dry-ass jambalaya. It wasn't a dish—it was a hug. How can you say no to a hug from someone you love? You don't. You accept the hug even if it's a little too tight, a little too long, or even if the person smells. From that point forward, I never said no to food that was offered to me.

I thought, very consciously, that turning down a meal

from someone could lead to, at best, anger, and, at worst, intense sadness. This belief connected me to food in an emotional way that is taking years to undo.

I would learn even more from my mother that food is love. My mother loves to eat. I learned from her the irrefutable fact that if a southern woman truly likes a bite of food, there's an adorable food dance that they do. My mom does that dance better and more than most people. She does it *better* because she's a great dancer and *more* because she's the best cook in Louisiana.

Of course, everyone thinks their mom is the best cook in the world. But honestly, all those people are full of shit. My mother is uniquely gifted in the art of not just cooking, but curating a meal. Not only can my mom cook and bake better than anyone, but she actually ORDERS and puts food together better than most people.

My mother is also a HEAVY cooker. And I don't mean just in frequency, but also in substance. When my mother makes a macaroni and cheese, it's heavenly. But I'll only eat my mother's mac and cheese once every two years. This is a pact I made with myself a long time ago. I came up with this rule because this dish is DEATH. It contains—and I'm not kidding—two sticks of butter, a can of condensed milk, two eight-ounce packs of shredded cheese, two fifty-slice packs of sliced sharp cheddar, two packs of cheese sauce, and bacon bits. And this is just a side dish, people. This dish is like a cheese-and-heart-disease goulash—and it's insanely good.

Having a mother who cooks like that is amazing. But it's also a challenge, because this is the person who crafts your first diet. During those first few years of your life, you're a hostage to that diet. Your diet is one of the most essential aspects of your life, and it's also one of the many things that you have zero control over when you are born. When you have a southern mother like mine, you simply eat what's put in front of you. If your mother gives you vegan or plant-based cuisine (poor child!), that's the limited option you get. If your mama specializes in yellow artery-clogging pasta and fried chicken, good luck seeing your abs anytime throughout your childhood.

But it wasn't my mother's fault that I ended up at 370 pounds with a blood pressure of 110/190 by the age of twenty-five. It was not. My obesity was learned, and my proximity to delicious food had everything to do with that.

When I was a child, my mother was always in the kitchen. It was a beautiful sight. There would be flour on her hands, a phone wedged between her shoulder and her ear, and she would be flipping or stirring something delectable. There she was, this godly being pouring herself into her creation. Seeing my mother in the kitchen could cure any ailment in my childhood. Is there a kid picking on you? *Have a little of this.* The girl you really liked didn't check the yes box? *Come taste this for Mama.* Before I knew anything about my mother's actual life, this is what I knew. She made the stuff that made me feel better. I didn't know her favorite song, the guys she'd dated before my dad, or what she thought about President Ronald Reagan. But I knew if she held out a spoon or a fork, magic was at the end of it.

I didn't know that food was an escape for my mother, too. Her dancer's body was gone. She sacrificed it for my sister and me. She'd leapt headfirst into the life of the homemaker and the caretaker. In a past life, she'd dreamed of writing words that would expose the plight of the liberated southern belle. That dream took her to college, where the bohemian lifestyle grabbed her. Experimentation of all kinds became her mantra. She once told me she felt free and unchained in college. My mother was certain that Paris, New York, and Los Angeles were in her future. But one day, at a gas station, she met a man. Then she put on a ring and birthed a couple of children, and that huge world became smaller. She was no longer the star in her own dreams. She took that same expression and experimentation, and she now confined it to one room. (Maybe another room, too, but I don't want to think about that.)

As much as Mom loved to eat, she rarely ate with us. She'd make a little side meal for herself and sometimes eat it while she was cooking. But as far as plating food for herself and sitting down with the rest of the family, she hardly ever enjoyed a meal like that. She would just watch. This woman who'd just toiled over gumbo, étouffée, or deer-sauce piquant would sit in a chair with a drink, rest her chin in her hands, and gaze at the rest of us devouring her latest creation. I feel like it was in these little moments that she made peace with the life she'd chosen. She and my father didn't have a perfect marriage (they divorced when I was twenty-two), but you could tell these moments mattered.

In all my years of eating my mother's food, she never, ever, ever cooked a bad meal. She's batting a thousand, and I suspect it's because she didn't want to rob herself of her peace. Like all southern Black women, she's impossible to lie to. If she'd bricked a meal, it'd be on our faces. She didn't want to live with that. She gave us pleasure in food, always. She solved problems with it and made our days better with it. My mother made promises to deliver it, and she always kept those promises. The lesson I learned from my mom is that food is COMFORT and PEACE. I've personally witnessed people reassess what good means to them after one tasting of what my mother throws down.

One particular time, my boy Ian came to the house and my mom had made some gumbo. She looked at him, smiled, and said, "You want a bowl?" I knew what was happening here. She wasn't being hospitable; she was being vicious. What she really wanted was for him to know that he'd never tasted anything like this before in his life—and unless he came back for more, he wouldn't again. I watched as he dipped his spoon into his mouth and then paused. "Damn," he said.

His mother was a brilliant, beautiful woman who always made time to cook for her family. Her cooking was good, but in this moment, I felt sorry for her. Her plates would be second-best to her son's culinary mistress forever. What washed over Ian is something I know all too well. I call it the Taste Blanket.

The Taste Blanket is that comforting and centering feeling that shoots through your body when you eat good food. For most people, the Taste Blanket is something that they pull over themselves every now and again as something to look forward to.

But for me, the Taste Blanket transformed me into Linus from *Peanuts*. I ALWAYS needed my Taste Blanket. It wasn't

that it was the only thing that made me happy. Being happy
at nearly four hundred pounds wasn't in the equation. At
that point in my life, food was the only thing that made ME,
period. Almost anything I did was centered around a meal,
a snack, or a drink. Nothing seemed worth doing without
the accompanying Taste Blanket. Food was not just comfort for me; it was a companion that I felt naked without. I
can't tell you how other people came to be food-dependent,
but I can tell you where it started for me, and for me, it
started at home.

I wish I could tell you I've since found better compan-
ions, but that would be a lie. Food is the perfect friend. It's
there whenever you need it, it doesn't challenge you, and
your mama is a fan of it. It's also an easy thing to get your
kids to play with, and all you parents know that. Burger
King had these little sliders in the '80s called Burger Buddies. I was obsessed. Burger Buddies were so small and cute,
like me at the time. My parents knew that I was obsessed
with Burger Buddies, so whenever I'd get a little anxious,
they'd get me some. I'd be busy with my burger friends,
and my parents could take care of whatever they needed
to do. This didn't happen all the time, by any means, but
it happened enough that even as I write this now, I have a
wave of nostalgia washing over me. Basically, I still want a
Burger Buddy, and I want it now.

It's hard to divorce yourself from the feeling that food gives you—that's why I'm not doing it! But I try to think things like, *Instead of comforting yourself with that food that your mom used to make for you as a kid, why don't you actually just call her! You know damn well she wants to hear from you, and what's more comforting than hearing from her?* The point is this: The Taste Blanket was given to me at home, so it will always feel good. Adulting, though, is making sure I'm not just doing what feels good *to* me, but also what is good *for* me.

3

Being the Fat Guy in the Crew

Being the fat man in my crew felt like I was living just outside of a dream sequence every day. I lived with this constant dread that anytime I walked into a room, I would be the fattest guy there and everyone would be looking at me. I have a group of solid friends that, to this day, call ourselves the Player Proof Crew. You'd have to have been around Baton Rouge in the early to mid-2000s to know just how cool we were—or how cool we thought we were. In all there are six of us: Ian, Geno, Ryan, Bryant, Trey, and me. Ian, Geno, and Trey were in a singing group at the time that was very popular. They were our local celebrities.

Being the fat guy was particularly tough. First, I'm not sure how it turned out that all of these guys were thin. We're talking about five graduates from the Chris Rock school of nutrition and fitness; the average stats for the crew were around six two and 155 pounds. My friend group was my emotional home, but I felt like an outsider. It also didn't help that they were so popular. Wherever we went, everyone knew them. They were in fraternities, basketball leagues, and student organizations.

During our time together at Louisiana Tech, Ryan discovered that he was sexy. When we got back to Baton Rouge after our second year of school, I realized that all the other homies had found their sex appeal, too. Everyone had done well with the ladies in high school, but in our early twenties things got different. College was where the crew's reputation with women was built. My life was the exact opposite of what was happening for my boys. I was the guy that all these beautiful women would call when they were having issues with one of my homies. I tried desperately to hide myself in the safety of our group instead of allowing myself to be seen. During those years with my crew, I missed out on learning how to be confident. My self-image and self-esteem were so bad that I didn't have the ability not to take life so seriously. I was afraid of becoming the punch line of a joke. I was afraid to take my shirt off in public. *What if everybody starts looking at me?* I'd think. Most likely, I wouldn't have been the first fat person that they had ever seen shirtless, but it didn't stop me from plunging deeper into my insecurities.

I loved these guys then, and I still do now. I am the godfather to several of their kids, and they call me Uncle Van. My boys and I still talk all the time. But being in the Player Proof Crew was hard for me. It fucks with your head to be the biggest person in the room but still be completely invisible. Not to mention putting up with the jokes. I knew that my guys loved me, but if you think they were going to spare me the jokes, you don't know much about the minds of men in their early twenties. We were vicious to each other.

Somewhere around 2002, a Player Proof member's dad had some legal trouble. It was a big enough deal that it made the local news. I just so happened to be at another member's house when a news alert came on TV. Our friend's dad was pulled into a police station while he was yelling at the news cameras. This scene was every bit as hilarious as it sounds. It looked like a skit from *Chappelle's Show*.

After the news alert went off, my homie left the room. He came back shortly with a videotape. He put the tape in the VCR. I asked him what he was doing, to which he said, "I'm taping this shit when it comes on again, just in case he jumps stupid one day." He was telling me that if our friend ever went too far with the jokes, he was keeping a devastating weapon to make fun of him. This is how far we'd go. Family potentially destroyed? Get these jokes. Got an STD? Get these jokes. Your girl slept with another guy? Get these jokes. Whatever weaknesses you had, they were going to be thrown at you.

Around this time, I learned something: The better you feel about yourself, the more powerful you are. If you're smart, you can handle being dumb for a moment. If you're beautiful, you can handle a bad hair day. If you're strong, you can handle a momentary weakness. But if in any way, you think what people are saying about you is actually true, an insult isn't just an insult; it's someone snapping their fingers and removing all of your clothes. You're trying to cover yourself so no one realizes you're naked.

My vulnerability was pulled to the surface with my crew a few years earlier at a Halloween party. We were planning to go to a costume party at a club called the NightLife. The NightLife was the dopest spot in Baton Rouge. We would go every Tuesday night. I would go buy new clothes specifically to go to this spot, because it was fantastic. Even thinking about it right now makes me feel amazing.

While I knew it was a costume party, I didn't dress up because I didn't want that attention on me. I didn't want to be the Kool-Aid Man, Ronald McDonald, or Rerun from *What's Happening!!* When you're a fat guy, as big as I was, whatever you dress up as for Halloween, you're going to be the fat version of a character—you're the fat Freddy Krueger, the fat Jason Voorhees, or the fat O. J. Simpson. I didn't want to be the fat anything. I just wanted to go to the club.

On that night, I get to my friend Geno's house and I'm dressed for a regular Tuesday at the NightLife. I had on a sweater, my durag, and some slacks. When I arrive, all of a sudden Geno's mother pulls out a camera and my boys start parading out. Ryan has blown his hair out in a big afro. Ian has permed his hair, looking like a pimp. Geno comes out with a beret on, and he is the epitome of a revolutionary from the '70s.

I immediately recognize that they have a whole theme going. They all look great in their costumes, and they know it. When we get to the NightLife, I see that all of the girls in the club are dressed up, too. Everyone is in a costume, except for me. In reality, everyone was actually too drunk to even notice that I wasn't wearing a costume. People were coming up to me and saying, "I see the durag, the slacks, and the sweater—are you Suge Knight? You're giving me this whole Death Row vibe." I'd shout back with irritation, "I'm not wearing a costume."

Nobody was listening to what I was saying because they were too busy having fun. My boys were trying to pull me into the party, but in that situation, I opted out on myself. All I wanted to do was fade into the background and hope that nobody noticed me. I felt terrible. Here I was standing right in the middle of a club, but there was a whole different life in front of me that I was missing. I wasn't missing out on a life of being thin—I didn't know how to be confident.

One of my darkest moments had to be during a night when the Player Proof Crew went to New Orleans. I was sitting in the front seat with my boy Ryan, and my boys Ian and Geno were in the back. During this particular trip, we were driving around and we saw this beautiful group of girls from Xavier University. In my opinion, New Orleans has some of the most beautiful women in the world. We picked up the girls to ride with us, and immediately everybody fell into conversation. While my boys had the gift of gab, they would let me do most of the talking, because I would often impress the girls with my convo skills.

As the night went on, one girl and I were having the best exchange. She was beautiful in all her twenty-three-year-old glory. Throughout the conversation, she complimented me several times and said, "You are different than the other guys." I was thinking, *Wow! I'm really hitting it off with her.* Ryan elbowed me with a smile and encouraged me to keep on talking to her.

The conversation flowed to talking about the guys from Cash Money Records. At that point, Cash Money and its artists—Mannie Fresh, Lil Wayne, Juvenile, and Baby—were the biggest thing in music. They were certainly larger than life in the Louisiana music scene. The young lady noted that she and her girls recently ran into the Cash Money crew at a local bar, but she was turned off that they were making it rain with money there. She said, "All of those guys were stupid. I'd rather date a guy that I can really talk to." I was getting excited.

Just as I was getting amped up, Ian asked her, "Well, which Cash Money dude was trying to talk to you?"

"Unfortunately," she said, "it was Mannie Fresh."

"Why is it unfortunate that it was Mannie Fresh?" Ian asked.

Without a beat of hesitation, she said, "Because I would never fuck a fat man."

As supportive and amazing as my friends were, they understood what had just happened. They knew that even though she wasn't talking about me specifically, she was shooting down my hope in that moment. But they were also a group of guys in their early twenties, so the entire car burst into laughter and I was destroyed.

This kind of situation with a woman was an embarrassment that I always feared. Now this fear had come to life, and I felt completely annihilated. She could see the disappointment on my face, and she said, "I didn't mean it like that. You're husky. I don't think you're fat."

"Stop," I said. "You don't need to apologize. I promise you that it's okay." It was a weird performance I'd learned, to comfort people who had actually hurt *my* feelings.

That incident didn't just ruin the night—it was a validation of all of the fears that I had about the way that I looked and what it meant to be a fat man. This girl had validated it. Everybody else would say, "No, man. You're not fat. You're fine." That night, she made my hiding make sense.

I ended the night early, and after that, I knew that I couldn't go out with them anymore. I knew that going out, meeting women, and experiencing life like my boys wasn't going to happen for me. I made it a mission that night to crawl deeper into the hole that I was creating for myself.

It might seem like having a devoted and awesome group of friends would have been liberating, but it wasn't. They were like my brothers, and they always wanted me to be there. Being with them did make me feel loved. In truth,

I've never felt more loved and accepted by any group of people in my life. And I knew that their love for me was genuine, because there was no reason for them to be around me except for the fact that they loved me. Their love and acceptance of me at that point in my life made me feel like I was a part of something.

But as much as I felt acceptance from them, I couldn't hide from the truth. Every single day, I was measuring my self-worth against my friends and their priorities. In a group of alpha males, there is definitely a pecking order. In high school and college, that pecking order was based on how much ass you could get. When you're that fat guy in a group, and the group's sole sense of worth and identity is based on how many girls they can smash, you never learn how to establish your own personality.

It hurt me to think that other people thought I was choosing to be fat. I wasn't consciously choosing to be obese. But if you're obese or even a little overweight, people tend to come down on you twice as hard. People will look at your excess weight and ascribe weakness to all different parts of your life. If you listen to other people long enough, when you internalize all of this noise, they will have you thinking you are emotionally and physically weak. It's hard to live in a world where you are constantly dehumanized.

People who aren't overweight don't understand the pain

of wanting to crawl inside of your own skin. And whether you just had a baby, are going through grief of some sort, or are dealing with extra pounds because we've all been sitting at home during the coronavirus, it's hard to tell somebody who is superfit how mentally challenging and taxing it can be to feel that you're not in the right body.

You might be thinking, like I was when I was younger, that just because my boys were getting all the girls they were happy. I found out years later that some of them were miserable as fuck. You're out here believing that your favorite girlfriend with the snatched waistline and the big smile on her face is living her best life, but you have no idea what goes on behind her closed doors each night.

It's insulting for someone who has healthy fitness habits to look at you and to tell you to eat less and move more. That's the easy part of the equation. But this right here? This is the hard part, feeling like the fat man out of your crew, feeling like the girl in your squad who is undatable and unlovable. This is the point in your journey where you have to stop measuring yourself against your friends and your loved ones and you have to get truthful with yourself.

4

Tyson Beckford Is a Lie

(Or How I Learned I Was Never Gonna Have a Six-Pack)

When I was about nine years old, I remember watching a Mike Tyson fight with my family, and my mom saying, "Wow, when Mike Tyson jumps, don't nothing move on him."

Dad looked at Mom admiring Tyson's body on the screen, and he immediately got pissed. "So what's that supposed to mean?" he said. "I used to look like that, but that body is twenty years old. Ain't nothing on him supposed to move."

This was the first time I realized that my mom could "see" guys other than my dad. They got into a long argument about that comment. I don't think that Mom thought Mike Tyson was particularly handsome, but she did recognize that he was built like a god. This was also the first time in my life I realized that you're not supposed to be fat.

I knew that certain people were fat and certain people were thin. I understood that different people had different bodies. But seeing my mom admire Mike Tyson's body and my dad having a very visceral reaction made me start to think about my own body. Throughout my childhood, my father used to refer to me as a Cujon. *Cujon* was a Creole word for "husky" or "fat." It's so interesting the way that country fellas can break you down anatomically and tell you what they think you are built and bred for. They'll talk about you like they're auctioneers sizing you up for the auction block. My father would always say, "You're going to be a big man, son. Look at your thighs. Look at the back of your neck."

As I continued to grow in my teenage years, my father would proudly say to anyone listening, "Look at the size of my boy! He's a Cujon!" My father took pride in me being six three and 260 pounds by the time I got to my sophomore year of high school. But his pride didn't stop me from comparing myself to men like Mike Tyson and thinking, *What do I have to do to look like that?* I started taking sports seriously and putting extra hours on the basketball court. I miraculously lost about fifty pounds. And as I started focusing in on my body more, I found myself going back to my mom's words and evaluating what was moving on my body and what wasn't. Everything was always moving.

As I entered my third year of high school, my standard evolved from one Tyson to another: the model Tyson Beckford. My sister had a famous '90s Ralph Lauren ad of Tyson on her wall where he is rising out of the water shirtless. Every time she and her friends got together in her room, I could hear them fawning over the poster. The more I listened, the more I recognized that they were NOT fawning over me.

This was an important tipping point for me as a teenager. I could have been logical and said, "Okay, they like him, but they could also like other guys like me." But that is certainly not where my mind went. If girls were fawning over Tyson Beckford, I thought, it was either that or nothing. When you're a Cujon-built boy in the South, there's only so much you can do to alter your body outside of genetics and sports. I was never going to look like Tyson Beckford, but that didn't stop me from obsessing over that picture and spiraling into a dark place about my body and who I was becoming.

The summer between my senior year of high school and my freshman year in college, I gained about fifty pounds. I was anxious and overwhelmed about my body, but I found some solace that my best friend, Ryan, and my first love, Paulette, were coming with me to Louisiana Tech in Ruston, Louisiana, about three hours from our hometown.

When I arrived on campus, it initially felt amazing. Paulette and I finally had privacy. We had the best bad college sex that you could have as teenagers. We didn't leave my room for the first four days. (Oh, to be kids again!) Ryan and I finally had independence from our really intense dads. Everything was great. But it didn't take long for my bubble to burst. As I mentioned earlier, this is when Ryan somehow figured out that he was sexy. He began making his way through the coeds on campus at a rate that would make Leonardo DiCaprio say, "Bro, slow down." Paulette was on a track scholarship, and her schedule was more demanding than I'd expected. And then to add insult to injury, I remember walking into her dorm room, and there it was: that same fucking picture of Tyson Beckford on her wall. Even at Tech, I couldn't escape feeling like I was never going to be good enough.

Looking back on it, my problem was the metric. All the mess was in the metric. I was judging myself and my worth solely on my physical appearance. Nothing else. Got a new job? *So what, you're fat.* Got a good grade? *So what, you're fat.* I was away from home, nervous about the new people I was meeting, and unsure if this place was the right place for me to be. While both Ryan and Paulette were learning new ways to shift gears, I was stuck in neutral, looking in the mirror and fearing the time that would come when I'd have to go it alone.

Not long after that, Paulette wanted her freedom. I totally understood it. All the guys on the track team had bodies that rivaled Brad Pitt in *Fight Club*. In a very short time, I lost my best friend and my girlfriend. I started filling that void with something amazing that I discovered in the Louisiana Tech student center. It was a hidden gem that only I knew about. It turned out that the student center had the best chicken tenders on this blue ball we call Earth. The chicken tenders came in a food boat stuffed inside a white paper bag. But, really, the boat was useless. There were so many chicken tenders and so many seasoned fries in one serving that a boat would capsize when filled with them. The bag was its saving grace. These chicken tenders became why I loved my freshman year at Tech. It actually became a running joke among people who knew me. As they would head to parties, study groups, and fraternity meetings, I'd say, "I have a date with CT—my chicken tenders."

When I lived at home and relied on my mom's cooking, there was a built-in control factor involved. She'd say things like, "Van, you've had enough." At Louisiana Tech, for the first time, it was all on me. I was armed with a meal card, a delicious distraction, and a fresh case of loneliness. I started to look at the chicken-tender window like it was my mother's kitchen. I planned my day around grabbing food there. I prioritized having some chicken tenders and carved out times when I could get them hot. After a while, I didn't even miss Paulette. I was nineteen years old and embarking on a period in my life where everything came second to food.

Then something happened at the beginning of my sophomore year. Aramark, a worldwide food-services giant, took over breakfast, lunch, and dinner for the student union. And then they did the un-fucking-thinkable: They got rid of the chicken tenders.

I remember a friend of mine saying that it sucked we didn't have the chicken tenders anymore but how great it was that we now had waffle makers. I lost it. Who wants a fucking waffle? Fuck a waffle. We had something that was THE BEST thing in the world, and I relied on it. I was going through a tough time in my first two years of college. It was full of ups and downs, both as a student and as a young man, but I'd had a constant. I had something I could turn to when everyone else was too busy, too sad, too horny, too tired, too preoccupied, or too unwilling to deal with me. And now it was gone. It wasn't coming back, and I had to find another way to fill the hole.

I didn't smoke weed or drink at the time, so food was the only thing to give me any kind of comfort. There was so much emotionally to deal with—more than at any other time in my life, because I'd lost my crew—that food was the only thing I could really count on. It was my best friend.

Toward the end of my sophomore year, I discovered a place not far from campus called Griff's. It was late at night, and I was very upset. The student center was closed, and I ended up at Griff's because it was open superlate. It was your typical greasy spoon that sold things like hamburgers and pork chops. When I walked into Griff's, I just wanted to feel that moment of bliss right before you start eating. You've done all the work to get there, you're sitting down, you're stationary, your body is ready for it, and you smell the food before it has even arrived. Food made me feel good to be alive. It gave me purpose.

On that particular night, I ordered a pork-chop sandwich, and it was disgusting. The experience got worse from that moment, because I kept eating it, and I knew that I was purposefully overfeeding myself—and that never feels good. I had a tremendous feeling of guilt about why I couldn't stop myself from overeating. When I got back to my room, I cried and threw up.

That summer, I gained another sixty pounds. I was packing on weight, and I was officially a big boy. My relationship with food became even more intense, and my weight continued to balloon. By the time I went back to Tech, I was well over three hundred pounds.

I can see now that I packed on all those pounds in college because I had too many transitions and not enough consistency. I wasn't prioritizing my health. I was looking to other things to keep me sane. And let's just be honest: That time after high school is a time when a lot of people start to put on weight. So if you packed on the Freshman 15, 20, or even 60, you're not alone. Yet I continued to hold myself to an impossible standard that I was never going to meet; I was never gonna look like Tyson Beckford, but I'd mercilessly beat myself up with guilt for not being able to achieve a body that it just wasn't in my genes to have.

I held on to this mentality until I moved to LA and met my friend Jesse Williams. I met Jesse on the basketball court at a gym in La Cienega, a little before he became the heartthrob actor on *Grey's Anatomy*. It was like the picture of

Tyson Beckford literally jumped off the wall. Jesse was a fully embodied person, though. Here was this really handsome guy who was right beside me, in flesh and blood, playing basketball with me. He wasn't some '80s cartoon villain. He wasn't a '90s R&B singer crooning about stealing your girl. Jesse was just a really great fucking guy.

Before then, I had this whole idea that anybody that looked that good was going to swoop in, steal your girl, and just be a dick. But Jesse and I met up on the court, he would talk with me about destroying white supremacy and shit—interesting stuff. After a while, we started playing a couple of games per week. Jesse would say things like, "Good shot!" or "That was a nice block, man." I discovered that he was really a good dude. And I started thinking, *Wait, am I becoming friends with this dude?*

If I'm being honest, when I first saw him on the basketball court, I'd wanted to destroy him in hoops. I wanted to destroy everyone, but this was special. I wanted to especially punish him 'cause he was a pretty boy. Men don't often talk about this, but competition is the best way for us to work out our insecurities. If a dude comes into the gym with something you feel like you don't or can't have, you go hard at him, let him know there's at least one spot where you got him.

This isn't just me, I promise. There's an example in one

of the greatest films ever made, the early-'90s classic *New Jack City*. In the movie, Wesley Snipes plays Nino Brown, the Center of the Cash Money Brothers, a New York drug organization. During the movie, the CMB is infiltrated by the FBI, with the help of a character named Pookie, played amazingly by Chris Rock. When Pookie's cover is blown, Nino's right-hand man, Gee, decides to blow up their headquarters at the Carter Apartments to burn all the evidence. Nino is obviously pissed when he gets this news. He calls a late-night meeting at his mansion to address how sloppily things are being run. During the meeting, he's using a slick black walking cane to point at people. Then he pulls a blade out of the walking cane and stabs one of his lieutenants in the hand, which freaks the fuck out of everyone.

The guy he stabbed, Kareem, was played by an R&B singer named Christopher Williams. Williams had had a hit with "I'm Dreamin'," and was the type of Black dude late-'80s women went nuts for: a light-skinned guy with curly hair. I remember that my mother and sisters fucking loved the guy. After Nino stabbed Kareem, he choked him with a chain. When they finally restrained Nino and pulled him off the guy, he looked at Kareem and said, "Never liked you anyway, pretty motherfucker."

Nino was the *leader* of the biggest drug operation in NYC, but he was still jealous of a dude he thought was better-looking than him. So much so that when it was time to take his anger out on one of the crew, he chose Kareem. Put the pretty boys through pain. That's what we all want to do. Until they end up being cool as shit. Now you're the asshole.

You'd think that I'd be used to this dynamic, being that my best friends back in Louisiana were so good with women. It's hard. Once you get used to fighting to be seen, it's hard to turn it off.

In LA, Tyson Beckfords don't just live on the wall, they are all around us every day. There was no way I was going to avoid being around men with six-pack abs and that perfectly cut V at the bottom of their abdomen. I had to find my own definition of how to feel good about my body, and explore what kind of body I wanted to live in.

You're doing yourself no favors by comparing yourself to the latest Instagram model. It's your job to figure out what your best version of YOU is—not some version of you that you think you should be. The journey is about finding the balance in your life that's going to make *you* happy. I was never going to be happy trying to fit into the Tyson Beckford standard. But I did discover what the best version of me was by figuring out what kind of Van I wanted to be.

UNLEARN OR BURN

5

Black Thighs Matter

Can you be fat, Black, and happy? I have asked this question myself a lot lately. As I write this chapter in the summer of 2021, I'm 280 pounds. That's a full 35 pounds heavier than I was before the pandemic. At this point, I know my body. I'm all right at 250 pounds, slightly sexy at 240 pounds, and Michael B. Jordan at 230. I'm discovering that 280 is interesting. While I'm still 90 pounds away from my heaviest weight of 370, I am still miserable.

I just can't think myself out of the fact that I'm failing my body.

What's worse is that I know *why* I gained weight. During the pandemic, my anxiety kicked into depression, and depression robbed me of my sleep. The insomnia was horrible. I wouldn't wish it on my worst enemy. Insomnia was like being held prisoner by my body. Sleep deprivation was like being on fire. I walked around all day feeling like my blood was being boiled on the surface of my skin. The worst part was that everything felt muted. My body was off-kilter, and because of it, everything else was off, too. I remember walking in downtown Los Angeles and seeing a homeless man as he was sleeping. Normally, I'd pity this man to the point that I would feel guilty about it. But not this day. This day, I envied him. Right there on that sidewalk, for that moment, I wanted to trade places.

After a while, my psychiatrist suggested I try a sleep aid. The first one I tried didn't work, so he suggested we switch to a drug called Remeron. Remeron restored my sleep instantly. The first night on Remeron, I slept eleven hours. However, there were side effects, such as intensely vivid dreams and being tired into the next day. One side effect that took me a little while longer to get hip to was weight gain. Three weeks into my Remeron usage, I'd gained fifteen pounds. Six weeks after I started it, I'd gained thirty. My doctor had warned that there'd be some weight gain, but I didn't expect this. This was like I was on a Krispy Kreme diet, with a Coca-Cola liquid regimen. I spoke to my doctor about it, and he tried to wean me off the Remeron. Immediately, I stopped sleeping again. I was dejected. I thought I'd made enough progress to stop needing a sleep aid. The realization that I was still at square one was tough to take. I was also really torn about my weight. I came off the Remeron for fourteen days, and in that time, I lost eleven pounds. It seemed like an impasse: Should I try to sleep or be slim?

Of course I chose sleep. Both my psychiatrist and my therapist have tried to convince me to not be hung up on my weight as I deal with my anxiety and depression, but they're not the ones buying new clothes. They care about me, but at the end of the day, they aren't me. So, now that I've chosen sleep, the question remains: Can I be fat and happy? Have I made losing weight too much a part of my identity? If, for whatever reason, I had to stay this size—or get bigger—could I handle it?

I remember the moment I hit the scale after starting Remeron and discovered the bad news of my weight gain. It was after the 2021 Super Bowl. My fiancée, Khalika, and I had gone to my friend Tommy's house to watch the game, and I ate like a pig, as most Americans do during the game. When I got home, I did this self-abusing thing I do where I weigh myself right after I've had a particularly bad run of eating. I suppose a lot of us do this to see what the damage is. When it read 280, my soul sank. I'd been able to keep my weight around 235 pounds for years, but now I was back to being nearly a 300-pounder. It had been a slow but deliberate journey, but I was back there.

The number automatically became my identity, and it couldn't have happened at a worse time. The pandemic meant that there were a ton of people I hadn't seen for many months. Now, it felt like when I saw those people again, they wouldn't really be looking at me. They'd be introduced to a past version of me, someone who I really thought I'd put behind me forever. Someone uncomfortable in their clothes, someone worried they take up too much space or that they sweat too much. I actually wasn't sure how I was going to navigate it. I felt intense anxiety around the idea of seeing someone I hadn't seen in a while. And I'm still dealing with all of this while my industry—one that requires me to be on television—is coming back alive. I hope to slim down, but the question remains: What if I can't?

I see so many amazing body-positive people in the world, and it's so inspiring. While most people envy the celebrities and athletes who seem to be cranked out from the perfect-body factory, I am superjealous of another group of people. I envy the ones who are comfortable in their own skin. I joked earlier about feeling like Michael B. Jordan at 230 pounds. That's kind of a lie. You see MBJ with his shirt off all the time, but for me, even at that weight, you'd never see it.

Most times, my body image makes me feel uncomfortable being seen. The most glaring example of this was right after my now-infamous TMZ encounter with Kanye West, when he told me that slavery was a "choice" and I told him that while he was entitled to his opinion, I was disappointed and appalled by what he'd just said. I went toe to toe with one of the most famous men in the world, and I had a moment that inspired a lot of people. But the very first thing I remember thinking when I saw the video was, *Damn. I really have to lose weight.* I was around 250 pounds when that happened. Everyone else was talking about what I'd said and who I was, and I was transfixed by how I looked. I immediately turned it up in the gym and lost fifteen pounds.

I've been taught for decades how to hate the fluffy version of me. I'm obviously not alone here. I've watched notable people, amazing people, deal with their weight issues publicly for years. When I was a kid, my mother, along with the rest of the country, would watch *The Oprah Winfrey Show*, way before it became a celebrity-interview vehicle. This iteration of the show was topical, and no one wanted to miss it. At the height of the show, *Oprah* averaged forty-two million viewers a week. I remember seeing my mom and a friend watching *Oprah* one day; they were completely enthralled with whatever was on the screen. Then, out of nowhere, my mother's friend says, "Why don't she lose some weight? With all that money she making now, why she wanna look like that?"

This was the first time I'd heard someone get at Oprah about her weight. I'd go on to watch this become a huge topic on her show in the coming years. Oprah, one of the most talented human beings ever, had to live out her body-image issues in front of the whole nation. She'd devote shows to weight loss and talk openly about her struggle with the number on the scale. It was sometimes as if every show had a subplot about Oprah's weight.

This comment was different for me, though. This criticism of Oprah's waistline didn't come from some soulless magazine or from an anonymous internet troll. This was from a lady who was my mom's friend and who made me lemon pies. From that moment on, I stopped looking at Oprah like a titan of pop culture. She was a fat lady now. Fat lady overrode everything else. To me, Oprah became someone who couldn't control herself. No matter what she did, it would be second to the fact that she was fat. Once *I* gained weight, it was hard for me to see myself as anything other than fat. But it has helped to know that it isn't just me who is dealing with this; Oprah's weight has yo-yoed over the years, and she's been open about fighting the same battle that so many of us are in.

The reality is that weight is just as big of an American indicator as race. Now, before you cancel me, I'm not at all suggesting that the ramifications for being overweight and for being Black are nearly the same. What I'm saying is that both conditions render a snap judgment from people. Without even knowing someone or their circumstances, people feel like they know something about us. To some, *Black* might equal *hood, criminal, emotional, promiscuous,* or *dangerous.* All of these things are often used to tell a story. Being fat has its story, too. Words like *lazy, gluttonous, unhealthy, smelly,* and *nasty* all come to mind when people think of those of us who are overweight.

Having been both overweight and Black, I can tell you that sometimes being fat is harder. Being Black for me has been the privilege of a lifetime. It's like being part of an incredible cultural fraternity that I couldn't see not being a part of. Also, there are some snap judgments people make about me as a Black man that you could argue are positive. The beliefs that we are sex experts, athletic deities, or creative geniuses all fall into this range. Most of these are just fetishizations of Blackness that come from living in a society where whiteness defines your worth, but nonetheless, they are there. On the flip side, try right now to think about one good thing associated with being overweight in western culture. Try to come up with one positive thing that gives somebody of larger size something to feel proud of.

That silence in your brain is the realization that there is nothing. Body positivity is so beautiful because it's the notion that you are attractive, healthy, and worthy of being seen DESPITE what society says.

When I lost over 120 pounds, I was superproud of myself, but my pride didn't come close to the pride that others felt for me. *Losing* weight incites a different judgment in people. I saw it everywhere. My first trip back to Baton Rouge after I'd lost all the weight was a revelation. A friend picked me up from the airport and burst into laughter when he saw me. "Damn, nigga!" he said. "You didn't tell me you lost a whole fucking cheerleader!" Everywhere I went, I heard the same thing: "I'm so proud of you!" The only other time this many people have been proud of me is when I won an Oscar for the short film *Two Distant Strangers*. (Yes, thank you, it was as amazing as it sounds.)

Hearing people say that you're fat or that you've gained weight, when that's something you struggle with, is debilitating. You already fat-shame yourself every day, a hundred times a day. All the outside world does is reinforce the pain that you inflict on yourself. You might think you comment on other people's weight for the right reasons, like to encourage the person to get healthy. But be careful—you could be making their state of mind worse. Imagine you're having a good day, not thinking about the troubles and cares you have; maybe you saw a great movie or spent the day with friends. For the moment, you're doing fine. Then you bump into someone that you went to high school with and they remind you of the forty pounds you have on you by saying some slick, irritating shit like, "I see you eatin' good," *chuckle, chuckle*. That day is fucked now.

Listen, if you want to help somebody get healthy, that's amazing. But you're not a drill sergeant, and no one asked you to be one. Honestly, I can't tell you how to approach someone about their health. I don't know who you know. But I can tell you that saying anything even in the realm of a put-down is the worst thing you can do. Put some thought into what you really want to say, and if need be, ask permission: "Hey, I'm worried about your health. Is it okay if we talk about it? If not, that's cool." Knowing that you care might be exactly what they need from you. And if they give you the space, take it. If not, kick rocks—it's not your life.

I heard from everyone about how proud they were to know me when I won the Academy Award, how excited they were to see me achieve something like that, and how inspired they were. This made total sense to me. Winning an

Oscar is something that most people would do if they could. The question is: Why were so many people who weren't overweight proud that I'd lost weight?

When someone takes pride in something you've done, it's usually because they feel a oneness with you in some way. Proud to be Black. Proud to be American. Proud to be from Baton Rouge. Were the people who were proud that I lost weight proud because I'd finally become one of them? Proud that I'd shaken all the implicit judgments they had and joined the "regular" human club? A less cynical way to look at this is that they were proud because they knew how hard it was, and people can take pride in, and relate to, anyone who does so. I can go with that. But I also sometimes wonder if the people closest to me saw me as Van or Fat Van.

I'm engaged now to a beautiful woman. Khalika's great and patient, and she takes no shit from me. These are all the things that I wanted in a spouse. I met her in late 2007, just after I'd lost weight. Like RIGHT after. A friend of mine, Jibril, had come into town and wanted to go out. I was relatively new to LA and still had no clue where to go. We ended up doing what people in their late twenties did in LA at that time, which was just roaming. There aren't really words to describe what being young, single, and out in Hollywood is like. It's electric, especially when you're new to the city.

The next night when Jibril was in town, we ended up

at the Standard, a supertrendy LA spot. We ate in the café there, then we went to the club, adjacent to the hotel lobby. I remember that Jibril had to agree to something called "bottle service" to get us in, and I laughed my ass off when I found out what it was. I called home and told everyone what a moron he was for paying six hundred bucks for a small table in a club. (We all later ended up becoming guys who would be willing to pay ten times that amount for a small table in a club.)

I eventually got up to dance as Jibril sat at the table and held court, because I'm amazing at that. And before I knew it, there was a sparkling Black creature dancing in front of me, then dancing *with* me. It's a connection that would last. There would be fights, there would be breakups, but here we stand. Still, I often ask myself questions: Would it have happened if I had been fat that night? Would I have wanted to leave the house? Would I have had the nerve to talk to her? Furthermore, would Jibril have wanted to hit the town with me? Which version of me is the world accepting?

Khalika would tell you that it wouldn't have mattered, and maybe she's right. But I don't know that, and frankly neither does she. My PTSD tells me that I can't go out into the world looking a certain way and be accepted in the way I want to, and I have evidence from my early days in LA.

Yahoo! Personals was a dating site run by, you guessed

it, Yahoo! It was hard to meet people in LA at first, so I created an account. This was a painstaking process. I was around 330 pounds at this time, and I did my best to hide it with my picture. I used shadows, angles, everything I could, and got what I thought was a slimming face shot, or as slimming as it could be with a BMI over 40. I accessed the most charming parts of my brain to write about myself, and then I let it fly. I just KNEW that someone would bite.

Day after day, I would check, and day after day, NOTH-ING would be popping. It was like a masochistic ritual. I'd stop by the fried-fish spot on my way home from work, boot up the computer, and then punish myself. One day was particularly brutal. I'd gotten a message from a beautiful woman who said she liked my profile and wanted to hang out. I hit her back, and to my delight she responded imme-diately. About ten minutes into the exchange, she asked me if I was a "professional man." I said yes, although it was a lie. I was actually working at an entry-level job for a video-game show. She then told me she was looking for a professional man who was interested in a discreet and casual arrange-ment. I was so country that it took me another twenty min-utes to realize she was looking for a sugar daddy. I had zero interest in being someone's sugar daddy, and I had no sugar anyway. My pockets were bitter as hell.

After that, I stopped checking the Yahoo! Personals

account. I never deactivated the account, but I stopped logging on. The next time I went on the site, I wasn't looking for love; I was testing something. After I'd lost the 120 pounds in the fall of 2007, I decided to update my picture to this:

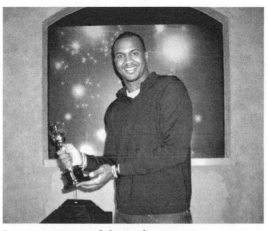

Image courtesy of the author

Looking at this photo now, I think I look relatively goofy. I don't have a haircut or a beard, and I'm not sure what's going on with my collar. Nevertheless, after I posted this picture, my Yahoo! Personals profile blew up. I had hundreds of messages. I'm not saying I'm anything special—just telling the truth of what happened. This confirmed to me that what I'd always suspected was right: There was a version of me people wanted, and one they didn't.

I now get to ask: What does taking care of myself look

like? Should I have done yoga instead of repeatedly watching the video of George Floyd's death? My father spent his
life stressing over the safety and protection of his family.
I'm spending mine stressing over the safety and protection
of an entire race of people. That makes the extra weight I
have not just cosmetic; it's actually life-and-death. It's the
difference between spending my sixties playing tennis or
spending them with a defibrillator implanted in my heart.

I doubt I'll ever have a perfect solution. The balance—the
peace of mind, body, and soul—is difficult to achieve when
I come from a place where people are always looking for
the next thing they'll have to do to survive. What I've had
to realize is that the journey to finding happiness in your
body has a lot to do with how healthy you are, and how
healthy you *feel*. No matter what readouts I get at the doctor's office, I don't feel healthy at 280 pounds.

My journey to body positivity will probably be a long
one. My question for the body-positivity gurus in life is
very simple: What if I honestly and truly don't love myself
as a fat man?

Is this something you can learn? If so, how do you do
it? Are their courses? If there are, do I even really want to
take them? Part of me is convinced the best version of me
is at 235 pounds, and I don't want to be anything except
that. Am I wrong?

Body positivity, at its core, should be the feeling that you look good no matter what the scale says. But real talk: That just doesn't work for me. I like how my shoulders look at 235. The way the skin on the bottom of my chin looks. How the veins in my arms look. How the back of my head looks. I like me, right there at that weight. Is that wrong? Am I asking too much of myself? I honestly don't know. I just know that, at some point in my life, I must reconcile feeling good with looking good, because you have much more control over one than the other.

For now, I'm in between. I'm not as big as I once was, and not as fit as I like to be. Is there a world where I'm happy with myself in whatever packaging I'm in? I honestly don't know. I know that I want to be healthy. I know that a big part of me wants to avoid the health complications that are common in my community. My own journey sometimes feels like a never-ending vicious cycle that I'm just keeping in check but not actually controlling. I've seen stress, diet, and environmental factors literally kill some of the people closest to me, so it's doubly hard to sometimes watch myself not have the will to avoid these same issues.

If you're like me, and you don't know if you can feel good about your body when you're out of shape, I have no inspiring words for you. I don't know if our kind is right or wrong. I just know that we seem unhappy and stressed-out while everyone in the body-positivity crew is living their best fucking life. They are on boats shirtless and in bikinis. They are twerking and twirling, and I'm watching every calorie and counting every mile. I don't have all the answers and I don't think that I ever will, but for now, I'm working my ass off to get back to my prepandemic weight—for me, for my future, and not for my Yahoo! Personals profile.

6

Depressed and Highly Favored

The absolute rock-bottom day in my life was when one of my producers saw me crawling up the stairs on all fours. By this point, I was working at Capricorn Programs, a TV production company in LA. I was on blood pressure medication and battling anxiety because of my embarrassment at being rushed to the hospital so much for my heart. I was closely monitoring my heart rate to make sure that it didn't spike too high. And I had taken to crawling up the stairs because I didn't want to risk the shame of someone seeing me winded—or, worse, having to be rushed off in an ambulance again.

I'd been suffering for years with severe social anxiety, an addiction to porn, and as many as three to four panic attacks a month. Some people relieve their pain with drugs and alcohol. My pain was coming out of my waistline. I was an overweight Black man from the South with too much time on my hands and no direction. I had no idea what I wanted or how I wanted to get there. I was stuck in a violent state of depression, anxiety, and food addiction. It would take me another two years and a humiliating moment on a GNC scale to finally take the first step toward changing my life.

My weight was my slave master. It dictated everything I could do, where I could go, who I could talk to, and what I was capable of. I took showers with the lights out. I crawled up the stairs. I ate alone so people wouldn't mock the fat guy.

Solitude became the way I coped with being disgusted with my own self-image. While it might seem like I was being too hard on myself, you'd be surprised to know how many overweight and obese people from all over the world deal with the same mental health issues, especially depression. A 1998 study out of Sweden found that "obese patients suffered from depression as intense as those experiencing chronic pain."

As much as it hurts for me to take in the truth of that statement, I also deeply resonate with it, because it has been my life story. I'm talking about a time in my existence when my blood pressure was 170/110 and my anxiety and depression required medication. In a nutshell, I hated being fat, but I also hated myself because I was fat.

So when the head producer saw me crawling up those stairs and asked me, "Van, what are you doing?" I knew that my weight was getting out of control. That very same day, I left the office and walked over to the nearest LA Fitness.

Now before you think that I'm going to tell you about some magical come-to-Jesus moment in that fucking gym, don't get too excited. My journey into the gym was a process that took me becoming absolutely disgusted with myself before I could even manage to want to try it. Unless you are living in a body where your self-image has affected every single part of your life, you will never understand how oppressive that feeling can be. I'm not just talking about the slight embarrassment of looking at an old picture and recognizing how much weight you've gained. I'm talking about the humiliation of getting on a crowded bus and you're taking up two seats. I'm talking about going to the barbecue and feeling all eyes on you because you added another rib to your plate. This was the gut-level humiliation that I took into LA Fitness with me the first day.

I walked in, and the first person I met was a brotha behind the front desk. I felt comfortable enough to say to him, "I want to start coming to the gym and get changed."

He said, "You're sick of it, huh?"

In that moment, I almost cried. I said, "Yeah, man. I'm just trying to do something."

I'm telling you, this guy was an angel. He read me right away. I don't remember his name, but he was the quintessential LA Fitness worker dude from central casting. He wasn't superlean, but you could tell that he worked out a lot.

As I waited at the front desk, he started getting everything straightened out for me. He hooked me up with everything I needed to know, assigned me a locker, and walked me around.

Then he said, "What's your phone number?"

I started to reply, "Two-two-five..."

"In order for you to get this discount, you're going to need a local LA number," he said, "so we're going to change your area code to three-two-three."

I was like, "You can do that?"

He laughed and said, "No, but we're about to do it."

This brotha was so committed to me transforming my body that he faked my phone number so I could get a discount. One of the reasons I've stuck with this same chain of gyms is because of this guy. We've all had that experience of walking into a gym and being with people who just want to make the quick sale. This guy was really showing me love, and he made it so easy for me to get in there.

After he showed me around, he said, "Well, you took the first step and came to the right place. Now, let's talk about your goals. What you trying to accomplish, big boy?"

When I say I was at the beginning of the beginning, I had no idea what I wanted to do. I said to him, "Bro, I don't really know, but I just want to lose some weight."

He was definitely the best person to get me started on this journey, because he simply replied, "All right, then, let's just start from there. Step one, let's get you on the scale."

The scale was at the front of the gym. Just as I was about to step on, this other guy behind me said, "Take off your shoes." I took them off, I saw the number, and I made weighing myself become part of my ritual every time I entered the gym.

After I decided that the scale would be the way that I tracked my progress, what made it even more special is that I would see the guy at the front desk every time I came in and he would be right there. Every time, he would look at me and he would be like, "Where we at?"

I'd be like, "We down ten."

"That's good," he'd say. "Keep working!"

A few months later, he saw me at the scale and he yelled out his usual "Where we at, fam?"

I said, "I'm down ninety-five pounds."

He replied, "Damn! For real? You got to let us put your picture on the wall."

I was feeling good, but I wasn't that confident yet. I declined, but it felt so good telling him how far I had come. He left the gym before I reached my goal weight, but I know I wouldn't have had the courage to get started if it wasn't for him being the angel that I needed at that time.

What was bad for me was that I was beginning my gym experience in LA. When you walk into any gym in LA, you're immediately going to see four things: an incredibly beautiful woman, somebody going fucking insane on a treadmill, someone else in an overpriced sweatsuit walking around taking phone calls, and a celebrity or three milling around in the background. When you see those people when you first come into a gym and you've never worked out, it's overwhelming.

Walking into a gym or choosing to join a new fitness class for the first time is scary as hell if you struggle with your weight, even if it's not in LA. I didn't even have any workout clothes. I walked in the first time wearing an old T-shirt, oversized wind pants, and shell-toe Adidas. And

I'm here to tell you that shell-toe Adidas are the worst possible shoes to work out in.

I gathered up enough courage there to start playing basketball again. There were a number of people who I admired at the time. There was a young kid who I would love to watch shoot and go through drills. I loved seeing him perfect his game. There was another guy, named Mike Lawson, who helped me get better with my shot. Every day, he spent a crazy amount of time perfecting his game, and after a while we started shooting together. What I didn't realize was that slowly my metric was changing. I was no longer concerned about finishing the basketball game. I now cared about dominating it. I wasn't exercising; I was competing.

I have always loved playing basketball. I still don't think I'm the most athletic guy in the world, but I do consider myself to be a good basketball player, with good hands and good feet. I played basketball all throughout high school and in different leagues throughout the city. Anyone who knew me from back in the day would definitely say, "Van can play." But at 360 pounds, basketball was not the easiest sport.

There was this ultimate asshole who I was playing with one day. I'll admit that I was playing him a little close and I fouled him. He didn't like the call, and he started going off. "Don't foul that fat-ass dude. He's not going to score," he said to the other guys. "Look at him. He don't know nothing about basketball."

This motherfucker had no idea how good I was, but with all the extra weight on my body I couldn't show him. I was embarrassed. Why would he bring up my weight in a basketball game? It was a small gym, and everybody knew that I was there on a consistent basis to get myself in shape. By that point, I had already lost about forty pounds. When the other dudes saw that I was affected by what he'd said, a few of them came to my defense quickly. The whole thing got under my skin a little bit. But you know what I did? I used it as ammunition to keep doing what I was doing.

I chose cardio as my first plan of attack, because I wanted to focus on losing the fat in my body before putting on muscle mass. I took on two forms of cardio to get my body going. I created a workout on the elliptical or an exercise bike and then I would hit the heavy bag. I also wanted to train myself to get into a regular routine. I knew getting a trainer or trying to stick to a rigorous routine at the beginning would be too overwhelming for me, so I started out by doing fifteen minutes on the heavy bag and fifteen minutes on the elliptical. To help pass the time, I would call my homeboy Ryan while I was working out. Out of all the guys in the Player Proof Crew, Ryan was the one who I felt most comfortable telling that I was trying to get healthy. I didn't tell everybody what I was doing, but he was the one who I knew I could trust.

At this point, I wasn't just in shape—I was in the best shape of my life. I was now 230 pounds and able to dunk like crazy. I didn't have a job yet, so I was playing basketball four to five hours a day.

One day, the asshole who broke bad on my foul three years before came walking into the gym with his brother. He didn't recognize me, because I had lost 140 pounds. I jumped on the court. I looked at him, and it felt like Christmas morning. We started off, and we matched up. I proceeded to bust his ass in every way possible. I was older than him but stronger. I wanted to reward my body for the hard work I put in by settling my score with this asshole. The game was for thirteen points, and I won by a score of 13 to 3. For the last point, I put him to the post just so he could feel my dominance. I wanted him to feel my balance and coordination. I wanted him to feel how strong my body had become.

Afterward, we dap up. He says, "Damn, I need to get in the gym. I need to get a little stronger."

And it was then that I said, "You don't remember me. We used to hoop over on Eighteenth Street."

"Damn," he said. "You were big as fuck, and you used to play in those busted-ass shell-toe shoes. Did you go to a clinic or something? I didn't know you had game!"

Basketball helped me improve my health and build community in Los Angeles. I began meeting guys on the courts during my games and it helped me talk and release some of my frustration and anger. Basketball became a way for me to not just be active physically, but also become active mentally and emotionally. Progress became my new passion.

I had to marry the fact that my progress wasn't going to happen overnight. I had to love the fact that it was going to be something that was going to take a little bit longer. I had to cherish incremental progress.

I had a basketball coach who used to have a great saying: *There's no such thing as a fifteen-point shot.* If you're down fifteen, you're not going to get it back right away. For me, I had to walk to the scale every day, knowing that it wasn't going to show me my goal weight. I had to do that for a year. The only way that you can do that is if your mind is different. Sometimes progress has to be the reward, and it's very hard to see that when you're first starting out.

I remember the first time looking down at the scale and saying, "Oh my God. I lost weight." I started seeing what was possible. I went from losing one pound to two pounds, and eventually twenty pounds. While all of this was happening, I was discovering that I could do a little bit more each day. The best part was learning that I could go from fifteen to forty-five minutes on the elliptical or the treadmill.

So I have a good routine in place. The pounds are starting to come off. My doctor takes me off one of my medications. I'm learning to like new shit like green juice and kale smoothies. And then—BOOM—there's some unexpected turn of events like the coronavirus, my fitness routine falls off—and I mean way off—and my weight creeps back in, and the anxiety starts, and the heart palpitations that I thought were under control come back into my life for the first time in years. When life comes at us hard, working out and eating right are often the first things to go.

So now I sit in body purgatory, not as huge as I used to be, but not as in shape as I once was. What does this mean? I have not a fucking clue. My perspective has changed enough to where I can't hate myself, which is a good thing. Still, though, I got used to being able to do some things that are a little harder to do at this size. I got used to wearing clothes that are a little harder to wear at this size.

I don't feel bad, but I feel different, and I don't know if it's for me. A friend of mine told me to love my body because it's the one that got me through the pandemic. That's fine, but what about after the pandemic? I'm forty-one now. Is it time to love my body as it is? Are my days of being a rec-league superstar over? What now? I honestly don't know. But I'll figure it out sometime during the twenty thousand steps a day I'm walking now.

7

There's a Shotgun Under My Bed

There's a shotgun under my bed, and I'm thinking about using it on myself. I'm thinking about getting out of bed, loading the shotgun, putting the barrel in my mouth, and pulling the trigger. It's April 2020, about a week before my fortieth birthday, and for the first time in my life, I'm not sure if I want to live. I think about the shot itself: *Would I feel it?* My fiancée would wake up and see me dead.

The horror she'd go through stops me. I breathe. I feel the life in me as my chest rises and falls with breath. I decide I want to do that again—breathe, I mean—so I do. Then some more, then some more, then some more.

The moment passes. I sit up in the bed and realize something: I'd just had a real, 100 percent genuine suicidal ideation. It didn't last long; all those thoughts seemed to happen in a millisecond. But they were genuine. I REALLY thought about it. The anxiety sets it—a rush of heat, followed by what feels like a pinprick sensation all over. My body feels it's in danger. My heart races; it feels like there are thuds and skips. It's a panic attack. I've had them for twenty years.

Careful not to wake my sleeping fiancée next to me, I get up, take all my clothes off, and go stand in the shower. For a second, I think I'm mistaken, that I'm okay, but then a second wave of panic hits, so I turn on the cold water and stand in it. The cold water washes me and provides an energy shift: relief. The water deshocks my system and recalibrates my body, and I feel better, calmer, but it's two thirty in the morning, and an ice-cold shower means my hope of sleeping for the night is gone. This is life with an anxiety disorder.

My therapist convinced me to turn over all the shotgun ammo I own to my friend and business partner Nic Maye.

I'd told my therapist of a night I was up all night long, staring at the wall, and wondering what the point of life was. I
couldn't sleep, I didn't have joy, and I couldn't look forward
to another day. The air felt thick with pain. I felt like it was
an effort to just get up and walk forward.

There's no good way out of that feeling, and there is no
magic bullet, except for belief. For me, this isn't a belief in
any deity or a mantra, but it's a determined belief in a future
where I will eventually feel better.

It wasn't until I was actually loading the cases of ammo
(we're talking three-hundred-plus rounds here) into my car
that I actually cracked a smile. I thought, *Yo, man, how fucking crazy am I?* When I got to Nic's house, he was waiting
outside. He took the ammo and was like, "Man, you good?"
To which I replied, "Obviously not." We both laughed.

I think back now to what my therapist asked me. I have
no doubt she was concerned I would hurt myself. But she
also made me complete a task. She made me confront the
feelings I was having. It was weirdly effective. My brain
told me that I wasn't well enough to have live ammo in
my home. My body then removed it. That entire time I was
wondering when it would be okay to have it again. As of
this writing, I haven't gone back to get it.

It wasn't until my first anxiety attack that I started to
understand it as going into warfare with myself. When you

talk to a soldier, the first thing they tell you is that a civilian can't properly define *war*. They tell you that because you've never been there and you've never been through it. They describe war as a sensory experience that Hollywood can't give you, no matter the budget of the film. Think of it as drinking spoiled milk. You can describe to someone what it tasted like, but unless they fucked around and drank the milk themselves, they'll never really know how disgusting it was.

I'll never forget when my uncle Charles, a Vietnam vet, saw me playing a military video game and heard one of the characters say, "Yo, throw a grenade. Clear a room. Switch weapons." I watched a silent rage grow in him. His body reacted with a rhythmic tapping of his foot, so focused and poignant the sound itself was almost violent. He adjusted himself in his seat like someone had turned a burner on under it. His eyes were locked on the TV. It was like the game had sucked him back into action. As if his body was reacting to being back in the shit after all this time.

Then out it came: "Y'all cut that goddamn shit off." He didn't say it; he yelled it. My cousins stood up quick and threw down the game control, stunned. But there was no talkback—Unc wasn't a man to trifle with. Unc then wheeled around and looked me in the face. "Van," he said, "it's not fun." He'd seen his trauma being relived as a pastime in this video game. It offended him. But even more than being offended, it reinitiated him. He was right there again, and it was like nothing had ever changed.

Anxiety is similar in this way. It's versatile and everywhere. I can hear someone talk about what it's like to suffer with anxiety, but I can never properly define their anxiety for them. It's not the same as mine. *Anxiety* can't be defined in an evergreen way, because it's different for everybody. The one thing that people with anxiety all have in common, though, is that at any time we could be reinitiated. The experience is so ingrained in us that all it takes is a scenario, a little push or tug, and we're right back there like Unc was. That's the common thread: the dread of reinitiation.

I didn't recognize that I'd had past symptoms of anxiety until after my first full anxiety attack. It's actually kind of funny. I could take one look at my uncle Charles and realize he was having a reaction to something, but I'd ignored it in myself. I thought it was no big deal to walk down the street and randomly think about getting shot in the back of the head. I didn't see an issue with waking up in the middle of the night in a cold sweat, or running into my parents' room thinking Freddy Krueger was chasing me, at fourteen. I never gave much thought to any of these feelings until they all assaulted me at once.

There was a state championship basketball game in

Lafayette, Louisiana, about an hour drive from where I lived in Baton Rouge, and my cousin was playing in it. Ryan—you know, my sexy closest friend—had gone to the same high school my cousin did, and we were going to drive over together. Ryan had started smoking a lot of weed around this time. He'd reached full Snoop/Tommy Chong status, where his personality didn't even make sense without weed. He'd become a living, breathing puff of smoke.

Normally, I didn't smoke with him, but we had a long drive, so when he passed me the blunt, I hit it. After a while, I just started freaking out. My heart started beating fast, and my vision got blurry. I was like, "Yo, you got to stop the car." At this point, we were in Breaux Bridge, still a little ways from the game. It's a sleepy town, and one that maybe wasn't ready for a weed-soaked 350-pound BLACK guy to be having a panic attack. But this is where we were, and this is where it was happening.

Ryan stopped the car, and I ran into a gas station and grabbed a bottle of water, and the lady at the counter is like, "Are you all right?"

"I cannot stop my heart from beating," I said, "and I can't breathe."

Now there were more people starting to surround me. These people were looking at my weight, they were looking at my size, and they went, "Hey, this guy's having a heart attack." Funny thing is, I kept waiting for my body to correct itself. I kept waiting for things to quiet down and for me to just be like, *What the hell was that?*

Believe it or not, that fueled the panic attack. The feeling that something is happening to my body that I can't stop or control can make me more scared, and away we go. Before you know it, there was a first responder there. He was taking my pulse and asking me if I could breathe. Like I said, this is a sleepy town, so the hospital is pretty far away. They called a helicopter. They never told me they were doing that, but I heard it. I heard a helicopter landing outside and legit asked someone, "Is that for me?"

More panic. More anxious thoughts. *If they had to call the chopper out, this must be serious. I'm definitely going to die in a place where they don't even have a Walmart.*

I got put into a helicopter and airlifted to a hospital in a different town.

Here comes the frustrating part about a panic attack. By the time I got to the hospital, I'd calmed down. But this would be just the first of several attacks that I would have that month.

On the following Tuesday, I had an anxiety attack while lying down in my bed with Khalika. She came home, we hung out, and it happened. I was rushed to the hospital.

That Friday, an anxiety attack hit while I was on my shift

at Best Buy. Paramedics came out, hooked me up to stuff, and said I was okay.

The following Monday, I had another anxiety attack, while downstairs at my friend Ian's house. It was the same group of paramedics who'd responded to my incident at Best Buy that arrived. One of them looked at me and said, "Man, you got to get a handle on this. There are plenty of things you can do. You want me to call somebody and get you a referral?" That was basically the first time someone suggested to me that I get help for my panic disorder.

With this new information, my life had suddenly changed. My anxiety was no longer an annoying backseat driver, chiming in when no one asked it to. It was now behind the wheel, with a firm grasp. I'd have to struggle to point the car in the right direction for the rest of my life.

Over the years, I've begun to recognize that some of my anxiety could be hereditary. And, in fact, the Anxiety and Depression Association of America confirms that anxiety disorders do indeed seem to run in families. Much like allergies or diabetes and other physical disorders, there is growing evidence that anxiety disorders can be hereditary and affect different family members in similar ways.

This makes sense when you think about it. Your parents are the first people who love you. The first people who care for you. Also, they're the first people who have the opportunity to fuck you up. They almost always take this opportunity, by the way. It's difficult not to. In order to keep you alive, they have to tell you—in great detail—what to be afraid of. Imagine what that's like coming from a parent who's afraid of everything. Angry at everything. Sad about everything. You don't have a fucking chance. In the community I'm from, breaking generational curses is like a lottery. We don't really work at changing things; we wait for progeny who are particularly talented or resilient to change the future.

My mother has an anxiety disorder. Like mine, it was hard for me to spot it when I was growing up. But after I noticed mine, I could clearly see hers. First time I remember it coming out was at a swimming pool. I was like eight or nine but already an expert swimmer. It was a beautiful Louisiana day, humid but clear, the type of day pools were invented for. This was the pool at our apartment complex, which meant it was *thick* with people on a summer day. Some friends and I were playing with a football. One side was throwing the ball, and the other side was making diving catches into the pool. Someone threw the ball to me, and it hit me in the head. As a gag, I went limp, acting as if I'd been knocked out, and fell in the pool. When I was swimming back up to the top, someone landed on me. It was my mother. She grabbed me and pulled me to the side of the pool and was asking me if I was okay and if I could breathe. I told her yes, that I was okay, but I thought it better to not mention that I'd been just kidding around. She made me sit on the side for a little while and watch everyone play. I was pissed about this.

What got me out of my feelings was that I noticed something else was happening. People were standing over my mother, who was sitting on a chaise lounge, and they were fanning her and telling her to breathe. I asked a friend of hers what was going on, and she said my mom was having a "spell." I'd freaked her out to the point that she'd had a panic attack. I just didn't know what to call it then.

It's likely my anxiety disorder comes from my mother. She's an amazing woman who gave me every ounce of decency I possess, and I wouldn't trade the experience of being her son for anything in the world. But, man, did she worry. Her worrying was the biggest point of contention between her and my father. She incessantly worried about everything, and he *seemingly* worried about nothing. My father once told me a story about me learning how to speak. For some reason, I struggled with *L* sounds, so instead of saying "look," I said "wook." Adorable, right? My dad thought so; my mother was terrified. According to my dad, she agonized over this. She spent hours and hours making me touch the top of my tongue to the roof of my mouth to make the *L* sound. He thought the entire thing was hilarious, because he didn't get why she had what he thought was an irrational fear. He did not get that she was wired that way.

From my mother, I learned how to obsess over what could go wrong. She always was waiting for the other shoe to drop, and now I am. I'm not saying that this is the ingredient that makes for a panic attack in you or everyone, or even in most of mine, but this made for an interesting dynamic for us. See, if I ever had a *real* issue, I couldn't tell my mother. I had to keep my worst fears hidden from her for *her* sake. We continue to do this dance today. I never tell my mom anything I feel is too big for her, because if she can't *solve* a problem, she *consumes* it. It becomes a part of her, and an unmeasurable weight. It's peculiar to not be able to share with your mother. It's peculiar to have to protect someone from something you know so well. I wouldn't inflict anxiety on my worst enemy, so I certainly won't give it to my mother.

What I did learn from my mother was how to cope. How to suck it up and get to the next day. She's a survivor, and she survives so brilliantly she makes it look like thriving. You'd have to really pay attention to see the pain. We still haven't healed, though. Her or me. We're pushing through and giving it our best, but healing is obscenely elusive. She's given me everything she possibly could have. Maybe healing is something we'll give each other.

My father had a different function in my life. While my mother tried her best to shield me from any potential wound, my father had the pesky habit of traumatizing me. One particular time was really fucked-up. It was the summer, and we were outside working alongside some of my uncles in the family cement-finishing business when my dad looked at me in front of all of them and asked, "Yo, you a virgin?"

Of course I was, but I didn't answer, because the question itself got such laughter that I was too embarrassed to speak up.

My dad continued. "Son, you a Lathan man. If you don't get some pussy by the time you sixteen, you an embarrassment in this family."

There it was: my manhood in one act.

So now, if I didn't have sex, I wasn't a man. And not being a man in front of my family wasn't an option, so I had to have sex. This now meant that girls weren't people—they were tools. Tools don't have souls. You can toss a tool and forget about it. Most importantly, though, you can always find a newer and better tool to do the job. With this narrative of not becoming a man in the back of my head, I was now placing my self-worth on having sex.

This fucked with me so bad, because it made every single conversation I had with every girl like game seven of the NBA Finals. If she said no to passing a note, that meant no to getting the phone number. No to the phone number meant no to the movies. No to the movies meant no to walking her home. No to walking her home meant no to going to her room, which meant no to sex. All of that meant I WASN'T WORTHY OF MY LAST NAME. Generations of men, Lathan men, were counting on me to FUCK.

These are guys who'd survived world wars, escaped lynchings, and built businesses. Men's men. Southern men. Important Black men. I didn't have to do any of that; I just had to convince one girl somewhere to give me five minutes. I started developing an INTENSE fight-or-flight response whenever a girl looked at me. By the way, they looked. I was a handsome kid, smart, and kinda funny (all according to my mom), so at some point the girls took notice. Because of this, I got into the habit of ignoring girls. Seriously. They'd smile, and they'd say hello, but I would pretend like I didn't see them. I was too scared to fail.

Obviously, my father and I never discussed this. That felt impossible. I remember I wanted to talk to him about sex once, and I even tried. We went to get po'boys from Rainbow Express. It was only about five minutes away from our house, so normally we'd take them home and eat them.

My father's truck was a work truck, so it always smelled like equal parts fresh concrete and fresh horses—not an ideal place to eat, until it was. He got in, turned on the radio, then began to fan the wrapping paper of the po'boy out on his lap. I then did the same. Man, this felt good.

My father is a lovable man, but not necessarily a loving man. I can't properly articulate what the difference is. I wanted his love and validation so badly that anything he did that showed me any degree of tenderness, I was over the moon. This was one of those moments.

I mentioned to him that some of my friends were starting to have sex (a lie) and wanted to know if there was anything I should know before I started (a pipe dream).

He took a pause, then turned the radio down. I thought "the talk" was coming. Instead, he said, "We got to take you to the drugstore and get you some zinc pills."

"What?" I said, genuinely bewildered.

"You tall. Sometimes when you grow so fast, everthang don't grow at the same speed. I ain't seen it, but your dick might be on the short side right now. Happened to your uncle. We get you some zinc, just to make sure. You know us Lathan men be packing."

He wasn't lying about that. The tales of my dad's horse cock had been passed around the family for years. It was a subject that made men joke and women blush.

I said nothing in this moment. I just sat there. Sat there and ate my po'boy.

So the question is: How do you get men—in this case, Black men—to not just eat the sandwich? To open up and discuss their feelings and mental health? It's simple (it's not simple): You have to create the value for it. Many people like to talk about how hard it is for Black men to talk about anxiety, but that isn't true. You just have to know how to do it. The first step is questions. We don't want the conversation to be weighty and built to be serious. You start by asking questions like, "How do you feel?"

I actually tried this with Dad a couple years ago.

My dad's response was, "What do you mean?"

I then asked him, "How do you feel on a general given day?"

He said, "Happy to be alive."

"That's what you *are*, Dad, not how you *feel*."

He let out a sigh. "I don't know. I never really thought about it."

There's a difference between asking yourself, *How do I feel, REALLY feel?* and *How do I WANT to feel?* I suspect there was a difference for my dad, because there damn sure is for me. I had an advantage in this situation: I knew who my father was.

His paternal grandparents adopted him when he was

a kid. He never really had a relationship with his father, because he was the result of sex outside of wedlock. Being the youngest of eleven much-older brothers and sisters who were actually his aunts and uncles made him binary: a teddy bear with the girls and a grizzly bear with the guys. His sisters doted on him in a way girls just a couple years older than him couldn't have. His brothers hardened him in a way that boys just a couple years older than him couldn't have. He didn't feel comfortable being too much of either tender or tough, so being detached became his thing.

Detachment was my father's trauma camouflage. It's the thing that he put on so you couldn't tell how much he was hurting. One of the most important things for survival where I'm from is how detailed and believable your trauma camo is. Be it humor, rage, lust, detachment, or any litany of things, what you show people to keep them from hurting you is just as important as who you are. Mine is humor, easy. Growing up, I'd make people laugh with me before they got the opportunity to laugh at me. That made me feel like part of the group instead of outside of it. As long as they were laughing, I was safe.

Opening up a mental health discussion in the Black community is like opening up a parachute. In general, you only open a parachute when it's necessary. Why would you think about opening a parachute on the ground? We have to repack all those feelings for nothing? Remember, discussing our trauma means our camouflage isn't working, and that's what's been keeping us alive.

All this means that once someone sits down with you to talk about mental health, especially a doctor or a therapist, it's going to feel yucky at first. Like, *Why would I want to talk about my emotional well-being with you? Who are you? And then risk looking and feeling like a total ass when I say something that you couldn't possibly fucking understand because you haven't lived one day with the shit I have to carry around all of the time?* As a whole society, culture, or whatever, we need to recognize that there has to be nuance to approaching, dealing with, and providing services for Black people in this country—and, in particular, for Black men who are struggling with their mental health.

Me and my boys talk about everything—every hurt, every pain, and every betrayal. But we NEVER talk about our mental health—not just how we are but how we actually fucking feel. We haven't known that we needed to. My homeboys and me have been wearing our trauma camouflage for so long that we can't even recognize our triggers. In my crew, there are womanizers, weedheads, narcissists, and liars, but not one of us knows how our behaviors were incubated.

Don't get me wrong—mental health is about the individual. Something that is this personal should be done on your timetable with people you trust. All I'm asking you to do is put on your oxygen mask. Don't wait for the progeny lottery. Don't be the one who can survive the punishment. Be the winner. Do the work now. None of us created this. But we have to fix it.

As Black Americans, we have to remember something, and it's painful: We didn't fuck our minds, but we certainly have to unfuck them. This is a basic human need.

We've been tricked to believe that a full belly is more important than a full heart. They're equally as important, and the hunger pangs from both are debilitating. One is immediate, and the other takes years to develop before it crashes on you like an avalanche. That avalanche has been crippling our communities for far too long. So I'm asking you to work on yourself, and I'm promising you that I am working on myself, too. But the work has to be done, or we and our future generations will suffer together.

Black people in America were handed what I call the triple crown of trauma, or the three e's. That's *emotional*, *economic*, and *environmental* destruction. Since we were brought here, our pockets, our homes, and our souls have not been safe. The very existence of Black people in America has been synonymous with the pain we've felt. And make no mistake about it: It was all done not just on purpose, but with purpose. The degradation of Black Americans has been studied, crafted, and instituted with a deadly precision for the intent of creating an intractable caste system that establishes America as a forever kingdom for white supremacy.

Every morning, you get to ask yourself, *Why do I want to be here?* For me, I want to see Anguilla. I want to see smiling children and frisky dogs. I want to see freedom. I want to see human inspiration and achievement. I want to feel my mother's latest recipe come to life in my mouth. I want to walk with Khalika. I want to create. I want to obey and disobey. I want to disrupt. I want to comply.

I'm making space to want even while I'm arrested in need. Admittedly, it's hard to balance the two when everywhere you go, you're reminded that things are askew. Seeing people wearing masks is a daily reminder. A mask is like a bulletproof vest for your face. It's keeping you safe, but wearing it is also a reminder that you need it. Wearing it actually means safety AND danger.

I've also deputized people as part of my self-care. For example, my fiancée can tell when I'm anxious. She'll ask me, "Have you gone for a walk today?" She once told me to shut the fuck up and do a puzzle. It's important to me that she knows what I need to do to get by. The people in your life need to know what you need—especially in uncertain times.

My deputies are my fiancée, my friend Charlamagne, my

therapist, and my dog. Khalika is the best. She has also helped to build me, so she can see the glitches better. I hope we're married by the time this book comes out, but I can't make any promises. When I'm out of whack, she's out of whack. When she's out of whack, it bothers me more than me being out of whack. At that point, I'm even more eager to get myself together.

Sometimes it hurts being seen and feeling naked and inadequate. There are times when I don't think that I need to have my coat pulled. I get lulled into thinking that I'm doing perfectly well and that I'm being my greatest self. I need someone strong enough, someone dialed in enough, and someone brave enough to tell me when I'm out of whack. Khalika is that person for me. Never trust anyone to maintain you who didn't help build you. That's one of the worst mistakes we can make. I trust Khalika because she has skin in the game.

As far as what Charlamagne has contributed to my life, it's as simple as this: Iron sharpens iron. He's an adult friend (a.k.a. a friend I made in my thirties). He gets where I'm trying to go and understands the things that derail me. He also struggles with his mental health. Having a friend who shares your mental health struggles is what I call therapy plus. It's a session without a session—and it's free. People in therapy tend to talk about their problems in a different way and with a different gusto. But I say, get as much free therapy with good friends as you can.

All that being said and all that being true, there's no doubt that we, those same Black Americans, have perfected passing on trauma. Black Americans have poured their trauma into art, sports, and the social movements that brought America out of its cultural adolescence. We've sacrificed our sanity to be the living, breathing beakers in which the American experiment is tested. Can people who were once slaves in a country see a time when they're fully free in spirit and in psyche? I say yes, though not because the forces against us will come to their senses, but because we will finally work together to control whatever it is we can. You might not be able to fix income inequality, but you can deal with your shit. Say it. Make the pledge: I WILL DEAL WITH MY SHIT SO A BLACK BABY DOESN'T HAVE TO. Taking charge of your mental health is difficult, maybe the most difficult thing you can do. For Black Americans specifically, there are so many things that challenge us every day, but if we fail to address the things we can, we'll never get the things we need.

HAVING SAID ALL THAT, I'M STILL FUCKED-UP

8

Lois, It's Kal-El, Can You Save Me?

One of my favorite people in the world was my uncle Markie. Markie, as he was affectionately known, was a good guy who was gentle, patient, and a gazelle-like six six, and who had the most vicious up-and-under move I've ever seen on a basketball court. Most people who knew him loved him and would do anything to protect Markie. When I first met him, he was in prison. I was around eight years old when my father woke me up one morning and told me we were going to see my uncle. Before this point, I'd only seen Uncle Markie in pictures. If you've ever known anyone in prison, you know exactly what types of photos I mean: groups of guys, arms crossed in front of some fixed background. Sometimes his arms were folded across his chest; other times he'd be squatting down like a catcher, or mugging for the camera with his hands straight out like he was going to give you a hug.

He didn't get out of prison until I was almost fifteen. The first thing he did was come to the house to have a game of basketball. We had a hoop in the driveway of our house, and a lot of kids from the neighborhood played there. I was already around six two, 230 pounds, so I could bully most of the kids that came around, and if you stepped on the court against me, I was going to smoke you.

Not Markie. The ass-whipping he put on me was legendary. He had a full array of moves. Markie was in his early to midthirties but was still cat-quick and wiry-strong. He outquicked me, outbullied me, and outfinessed me. He also coached the whole time. "Van, don't reach," he'd say. "You're out of position." Then he was gone, to the basket and above the rim.

He had played lefty the whole game, and I remember telling him I didn't know he was left-handed. "I'm not," he said, laughing.

My father had told me my uncle Markie was good, but my father's sports stories are fantastical enough to make Marvel movies look like documentaries. He was right this time, though. Markie was incredibly skilled. He'd jump by my right side, and if I didn't go left right away, he'd scold me. "You have two hands, big boy," he'd say. "Use 'em both, or you just gon' be a walking turnover." He decimated me in the game, but he managed to make me feel like I'd won.

After that first game, I talked to Uncle Markie for a while. I really didn't know much about him, and I wanted to close some cases in my mind. I began firing questions at him:

What did you do?
Why did you do it?
Are you sorry?
What was prison like?
Did anyone hurt you while you were inside?
Did you hurt anyone?

The answers came as rapidly as the questions did:

Armed robbery.
I was on drugs.
Yes.
Silence.

Yes.

Yes.

I noticed he'd skipped one question. So I asked it again: "What was prison like?"

He hadn't been ashamed to answer any of the other questions, but for some reason he was struggling with this. I saw a lump form in his throat. He pushed the lump back, then pushed the words out of his mouth.

"You're just stuck. You fucked up, and now you're stuck. You're stuck so far down that it don't seem like it's nothing you can do to get out from under. But most times, you can. It just seems like where you wanna be is so far from where you trying to be, that it don't even make sense to try."

I'll never forget the look on Uncle Markie's face after he said that. The experience of incarceration enveloped him like a poisonous shadow. He was free now, but he could replay his hopelessness like it was his favorite song.

It started with his hands, which began to shake as he attempted to dislodge a cigarette from a carton and light it. The smoke began to build as the shadow spread to his head. His eyes got sort of fixed on the horizon in a half stare/half gaze. The state penitentiary in Angola was at least sixty miles away from us, but it seemed like he was looking directly at it. Finally, the shadow took his body over, and he began to look around for a place to sit down. He just sat there for a second and said, "Damn." It was as if the thirteen years in prison that he'd experienced just hit him all at once.

Sometime after his release, Markie began to use drugs again. I recall hearing my dad complain, something he rarely did, that "Mark fucking with that shit." This was often accompanied by him admonishing me, "If I ever catch you fucking with that shit or bringing it into my house, I'll fuck you up like a grown man, you hear me?" My father was hurt about his brother's drug use, but rather than talk to someone, anyone, about it, he put fear into his son. He felt fear was the only weapon he had to keep him from watching drugs take me, too.

In South Baton Rouge, the drug of choice was crack, unless you had a little money and could afford to snort brown (heroin). We all knew someone, multiple people usually, who were battling it. It wasn't even a thing, it was just a reality.

Markie's use of crack led to an accident that would change his life. The story goes that he was in a hotel room when he tried to light a dope pipe. But, apparently, there was a gas leak in the room. When the lighter sparked, the room went up. Markie suffered third-degree burns all over his body. He would never look or act the same again. Occasionally, he'd stop by the house while I was playing basketball and I'd toss him the ball, and he'd take a shot, wincing while doing it. His body had been through too much. Eventually, I stopped tossing to him.

There was a settlement from the accident, which gave an addict exactly what he didn't need: a huge pile of cash. He never got control of his addiction, but he lived longer than we thought he would. He passed away in 2015. He was fifty-five.

I can't convince you that my uncle was a good man. And honestly I don't know if I want to. He was a felon, an addict, and sometimes a pain to his mother and siblings. But he was also kind. Uncommonly kind. He once asked me if they still did free lunch in school. I told him I didn't know, because we had a pizza station at lunch and that's where I'd get my lunch most days. He told me I was blessed to not need help from the government. He suggested I find a free-lunch kid and buy him some pizza one day. "Imagine expecting lunchroom pizza and getting Domino's," he said. "You'd have a friend for life, bless somebody."

My dad told me that was dumb as hell and that I'd likely embarrass the kid I was trying to help. He also thought that Uncle Markie's suggestion was rooted in some "jailhouse cafeteria bullshit," which could've been true. Still, I took it then just like I take it now: Uncle Markie had wished someone was around to buy *him* pizza when he was a free-lunch kid. No one is more appreciative of kindness than those who've lived without it. He wanted me to put more of it into the world because he believed I was in a position to.

When he passed away, I thought about who he could've been if he'd never gotten behind life's eight ball. I'll never know. He lived his life the best he could, but in the end, the beautiful and capable body he'd been given was beaten down and destroyed by the choices he made—and by societal choices that were made for him.

My uncle's death made me feel untethered. I was thirty-five when he passed away, and that's about the age you start to memorialize your youth. Your hair starts thinning, your knees start hurting, and you realize this body is temporary. It's breaking down in front of you, and you can see it. That made me think about the peculiar condition of Blackness. Black American life is as uncertain as white supremacy is certain.

That's what American freedom means to me: certainty, or at least the feeling of it. You call the cops, you KNOW they're coming, and you KNOW you'll be okay when they do. You KNOW you're going to get a good job; you just have to decide which one. You're getting that loan, you're getting that promotion, and if you don't, you're speaking to the manager.

My upbringing was totally different. I was told that catastrophe was ever present, and if I wanted to avoid it, I had to thread a very specific needle. If not, my future would be crime, prison, drugs, and death, just like Uncle Markie's. He never came out of it. There was no Malibu rehab stint. He didn't give his life to Jesus or Elijah Muhammad. He didn't *live*; he just *survived* for fifty-five years.

To Mark Lathan, everything was a gamble, and he doubled down until he doubled over.

Walking around as a Black man for more than forty years, screaming at the top of my lungs about the condition of my people, and the needs of my community, I'm fucking tired. The whole thing is exhausting.

Let me give you an example of this fatigue. As I write this, the whole world is mourning the death of DMX. X, born Earl Simmons, was a man not unlike my uncle Markie. He was gifted, tortured, and touched. To love X was to submit yourself to an experiment in the beautiful yet dysfunctional parts of Black American urban life. X was a devout Christian who always spoke on the virtue and redeeming value of Christ. Yet he'd been to jail thirty times, for crimes ranging from DUI to robbery. He was also an addict, and it's his drug use that ultimately took his life. His music was often homophobic, misogynistic, and hyperviolent, with some lyrics bordering on ghastly. Despite all this, we LOVED this guy. Like LOVED. There was a brutal truth in him that made us feel at home.

Now, I don't mean to speak for all Black people. Never do I want to do that. I'm talking about a general feeling, almost like a wavelength of despair. The reaction to X's coma illustrates the divide in the American psyche. Black Americans started praying, and it seemed white Americans started printing. I saw tweets about how recklessly X lived life. Think pieces about his legal troubles. The *New York Post* ran a disgusting article listing all the homes he'd lost during his career. All this while we just wanted to mourn.

So many of us just wanted space to be human. We understand the DMXs. We know them. We want them to do better, but at some point we take them for who they are. Watching people get their takes off his mishaps was just soul-draining for me. I took every shot at DMX personally. Not because I'd ever met him—I hadn't. It wasn't really him I wanted to defend. It was his humanity.

Imagine walking around all day defending your humanity. Explaining to people why other people matter. Explaining to people why we're turning the page on certain practices and traditions. Don't get me wrong—I LOVE being Black. But it's obvious that the rest of America DOESN'T love that I'm Black. If they did, they wouldn't take my Blackness as such an insult. These microaggressions, plus the real-world macro ones, like police violence, poverty, and environmental apartheid, keep me wound up, and that takes a lot of energy.

It may sound like I'm angry. But I'm beyond angry. I have a visceral and deeply rooted disdain for the American status quo. White Americans have a god complex. Gods get angered when you ignore them or defy their rules. You can't share a community with a god or a god complex. Communities need cooperation, not worship. Yet white Americans want to be worshipped. White supremacy has to be worshipped in order for it to exist.

When God created the heavens and the earth (if you believe in that sort of thing, which I do), he had just two demands of humans: fellowship and fealty. God wants you to acknowledge him and to honor his wishes for you. This requires praise, sacrifice, and trust. You do this because there's a fundamental understanding that without God, you'd be nothing. You'd be part of the vast and random void of space and time. God gave you fruit, sex, rock and roll, honey buns, posters, roller coasters, Sprite, beaches, the NBA, the whole ball of wax, life.

Believe it or not, white supremacists think they gave the same things to Black Americans. The notion is that we were wandering in the nothingness of a savage continent, and some white dudes scooped us up and taught us how to use a salad fork, then—BOOM—society. For this, it's demanded that we shut up and dribble. At the root of the white-supremacist ideal, anything we do is because the white gods have deemed it so.

This is another reason why we're so easy to kill. One of the first things any religion tells you about God is that he takes your life whenever he wants to. It's a fundamental part of the deal. God understands something you don't, is powerful in a way you can't comprehend, so the taking of your life only has to make sense to *him*. Does that sound familiar? Does that sound like millions of slaves 150 years ago? Does it sound like police violence today? Does it sound like flooding crack into neighborhoods to fund wars abroad? Of course it does.

By the way, the God complex is all a lie. You see, God built the world by himself, while the world we're living in, we built. We've had a hand in building America at every step along the way. The only reason we've not been recognized for our part in it is because we've been told to follow white supremacy's plan.

Here's the rub with everything I've just told you: The more you know, the angrier you get. The second thing I will say about Uncle Markie, other than that he was kind, is that he wasn't an angry man, just sad. He, like my father, lived a relatively simple life, and didn't really consider conditions as much as I do. I isolated myself from my family a lot as a kid for this reason. My father called it "fretting." It was very funny to him. "That boy always fretting about something," he said. He was right. Slowly, my fear became anger. And the older I got, the more my anger has caused depression.

I first noticed this during the aftermath of George Floyd's death in May 2020. Watching the life drain from George, I felt his face on the pavement. I felt the knee in the back of his neck. I could hear the sounds of people yelling. I felt the fear that set in as he realized that his trip to the store had become a trip to the hereafter. I watched the video of George Floyd's murder over and over again, and I'm not sure why. Maybe I hoped to see something that would make it make sense. But nothing did. Every time I watched, it just made me angrier.

I wanted to hurt someone. I wanted to physically make someone feel what I felt mentally. But I couldn't. It's not in me. I just had to sit with my anger coursing through me. I had no outlets to channel my feelings. I'd just sit alone—a Black man myself and still alive—pondering the point of life. *Nothing would change*, I thought, *and so what was the point of even trying to change anything?*

One way to marginalize Black people or to oppress Black people, or any group that's been oppressed over the course of the history of America, is to convince them that what they're saying isn't true, that we've had it just the same—which is a wild lie, right? We've been given nothing but pain. We've been punched in the eye and then criticized for bruising too easily. The older I get, the more I realize I can't change this. And there is a pain behind this feeling that I can't articulate.

There was a time in my life when I thought this generation would change it. This culminated with Barack Obama's election. I, like many others, was elated at the idea of a Black president, so much so that I ignored the very real hurdles, both socially and economically, that still had to be jumped for America to achieve any sort of racial harmony. What I've learned is that we'll likely never get there as presently constituted, because we don't want to. There are parts of America—large parts—that have zero interest in my life mattering at all. And they always will. The parts of America that do care about my life mattering won't help us fight for it, because that other part is their brother-in-law. Or cousin. Or business partner.

Black American lives are the currency in a white American truce, each side agreeing that no matter how bad things get for them, it could always be worse. White Americans could be us. Our true emancipation would mean the end of that truce, and I don't believe either side actually wants that. So instead, you get us: the descendants of capitalism's first and best mules left to wander in a land never built *for* us but built *by* us.

I think about that when I think of "listening to the other side." I think about it when I hear "Just comply with the police." I think about it when I see protesters being called traitors by people who build statues to actual traitors. It makes me feel helpless and angry, but also focused and sometimes violent. I often wonder just how much of my anxiety and depression is my mind reminding my body that it doesn't feel free.

When people talk about being divisive, it's because there's an intense amount of tribalism that is going on in every single cultural conversation that we have. Now, a lot of it is understandable, but that doesn't change the fact that if we're to get to a place that's better than the place we are right now, then we're going to have to find a way to cut through it.

Trust lives inside of humanity. Relating to someone on a human level is about trust. If we're talking about the killing of an unarmed young Black male or female, the first thing that everyone should agree on is that it's a tragedy, that somebody's mom is going to cry about it, somebody's dad is going to cry about it, there's a community that is going to be affected. The first thing that should happen is there should be a connection on a human level. If you come to me and you say "The thug got what they deserved," now I have to come to you and do something that Black Americans and other types of Americans have done throughout the history of the country, which is explain to you why this young Black person is worthy of life. I'm asking for people, in the face of tragedy, in the face of progress, to be a little bit more human.

Recognize, before it gets politicized, that somebody lost their life, and then let that spring you to trying to understand how we can stop that from happening. I think that with social media (which I don't see as the great evil that a lot of people do) the reaction to these murders is becoming cold and automatic, and the buzzwords come out faster than the healing does. The first thing that we need to do is just recognize that we're all people. That's difficult, I know. We bring a lot of stuff with us.

I've experienced a ridiculous degree of racism, so there's a latent distrust for mainstream America that exists inside of me. I've got to work that out for me, *for me*, in order to best represent my culture and my community. At the same time, that's work that everybody has to do. As Black people moving through the stress, the anger, and the triggers of racism and patriarchy, we're all in crisis, so let's treat ourselves like we are. It may feel like in order to see change through, we have to stop being people and turn into warriors. But warriors need allies. And if you can't rely on the ones outside of yourself, you can take the steps to become your own ally. My days are now about 60 percent self-care. I start the day with a morning walk. After that walk, I meditate and write.

That's what self-care feels like to me, a person who didn't give a shit about self-care years ago. *Self-care* was something that one rich white lady said to another rich white lady in a spa. It had nothing to do with me. Now I've learned to love on myself the same way I would love on a sexy girl that I was excited about taking out. In fact, this date is so fine that I pull out all the stops. This date is so important to me, as I've been fighting for more than forty years now for this, that I don't let anything come between us.

When you first meet someone, you do everything in your power to make their day a little bit easier. You ask them what they need, what they like, and what they want. We do that for everyone else, but not for ourselves. Now it's vital. As I write this, I have my diffuser going, mood lighting on, and Jay-Z playing in the background. It's a mood I've set for myself. This is the same type of mood I'd set if I was trying to get a little bouncy-bounce ass.

I'm not checking the latest news, I'm taking headspace from scrolling through the Black bodies being shot on my feed, I'm not watching the DC circus, and I'm not obsessing over the couple of extra pounds under my shirt. I've created a peaceful space for me today and in this moment.

Beating the racism, sexism, and inequality we deal with every day is insanely taxing, even for the greats. History doesn't often tell us of the extreme depression and anxiety felt by men like Martin Luther King Jr. and Malcolm X. That's not part of the story. The part of the story we're supposed to remember is that they worked their way through every obstacle to help create the freedoms we all enjoy today. So many of our examples were superhuman, so why can't we be as well?

Well, we're not. You're not superhuman—you're very human. We all are.

9

The TMZ Chapter

Everywhere I go, people ask me about my time at TMZ. During my last few months, I hated working there. I'd have to give myself a pep talk to start every Monday morning, or I would call friends on Sunday night to make me get up and go in. I wasn't alone in being frustrated with my job.

There are millions of Americans who could write at length about this feeling. It's one of the sadder things about American life. We spend approximately ninety thousand hours of our lives working, while I would dare to estimate that eight out of ten of us are dissatisfied with the places we work. People have all kinds of reasons they're unhappy at work. Some feel that they're underpaid, while others feel that they're underappreciated or underestimated. But more often than not, our work life includes being overworked and overstressed.

Where I grew up, people don't even attempt to be happy at work. Work is a place where you sell your happiness. If you are lucky, you might get a halfway-decent vacation or a good happy hour once in a while.

This cycle of unhappiness is exacerbated in the Black community. Jobs are scarcer, so if you get one that pays you a decent salary and values you, you're probably going to take a lot of shit to keep it. That economic insecurity exists for a lot of working-class Americans, regardless of race, but race certainly complicates the matter. For a lot of the people I grew up around, one pink slip could change their entire lives. I'm not talking about a momentary hiccup, where they're out of work for a little while and then back on the horse. I'm talking South Louisiana in the '80s and early '90s, where the unemployment rate was the highest in the country.

Things got so bad for finding a good job in my home state that my beautiful, amazing Louisianans actually flirted with the idea of electing a former grand wizard of the Ku Klux Klan as governor. David Duke told the white working-class people of the state that he was looking out for them, and that he'd make Louisiana great again. Duke's greatest weapon was, of course, race. He convinced nearly 40 percent of Louisianans that the reason why they didn't have jobs was because affirmative action had given all the employment away to the dregs of society, who were living high off the hog while they got left behind.

All of David Duke's campaigning was a fucking lie, which anyone with a shred of information and an objective mind could destroy. But it was still compelling enough to make some people put their long-hidden racism on full display.

As pissed off as I get rehashing this history, I understand those Duke voters now. I don't give them a pass for supporting unabashed and emboldened white supremacy, but being insecure makes you do shit and take shit that might not otherwise pass your smell test. Everyone wants to believe that in a moment of moral crisis, we'd put our integrity over money. We all want that freedom, although very few of us have it. So most people hold their nose and put up with the shit, forever.

I didn't take much shit at TMZ. In fact, most employees who worked with me would probably describe me as a constant line-pusher. I was important there, and I knew it. I'd become a fixture on three different TMZ television shows, and that meant I was due a little star treatment. This is not a thought I'd ever actually had or even verbalized only to myself; it's just something I knew to be true. I could come in just a little late, leave just a little early, and say things other people definitely couldn't get away with. I'd built this by being someone you could count on to deliver.

I began at TMZ as a tour guide. It had started a new brand called the TMZ Tour, and it needed guides. The tour was billed as a "show on wheels," so you'd have to be a host on wheels. We'd start off in Hollywood, then make our way to West Hollywood, Beverly Hills, then back to Hollywood, before finishing up at Grauman's Chinese Theatre. Hosting the tour was some of the most fun I've ever had at work. I got to be funny, informative, and the star of the show for two hours. Mostly, though, I got to do my favorite thing, which is to talk to people. People come to LA as tourists from all over the world, and after a while my job became learning about these people and what they were into.

We weren't contracted with TMZ as employees and made a pretty low base hourly wage. And when I say low, it was *low*. A tour guide friend of mine, who was an amazing guide, cracked under the pressure of the job. There was one tour where he felt particularly stiffed by the audience. Sometimes you'd kill it and they wouldn't give you a tip, and sometimes you'd phone it in and make two hundred bucks. This guide was pissed he didn't make bank, so he followed a guest to the bathroom and demanded his money. When I first heard the story, I couldn't believe it was true, but after reading on Yelp where the guest gave one star and a hilariously blistering review of the tour, I had to admit it happened. My friend the gutsy guide was fired immediately, and I was given his load of tours.

I started to feel like the whole tour was on my back, and I had to deliver to make it a success. This was a precarious time in my life. Before joining TMZ, I was unemployed for two years during the Great Recession in the late 2000s. Similar to Louisiana in the '80s and early '90s, if you had a job, you kept it, and if you got hired, you fucking appreciated it. I'd come to LA to work in film and television, and this job at TMZ was as close as I'd ever been to either. I dove headfirst into it.

One day, Harvey Levin, the head of the whole company, came to watch my tour. I was immediately asked to appear on the television show. This all happened in a blur. I went from being a tour guide to being on a nationally syndicated TV show in about three months. If you listen hard enough, you're going to hear bad things about Harvey Levin. You might even hear some later on in this chapter. Despite this, I have to admit I owe him a great deal.

The very first time I appeared on TMZ, he teed me up to have my moment. Harvey knew how tough it is to break through, not only with the television audience, but also with the other people in the room. The bullpen that you see on TMZ isn't just a group of television personality types. These are coworkers who work in different departments around the organization. We'd literally shoot the show in the morning, then go work on our various TMZ-related jobs for the rest of the day. For me, that meant shooting the show, then going to do tours for the rest of the day. It also meant that if I was going to come in as a new guy, I'd have to bully my way in. I was fighting for camera time with people who actually made the show, had known each other for years, and didn't really give a fuck whether or not my people back home got to see me on TV.

Breaking in at TMZ was hard, and Harvey knew it, so when it was appropriate, he had me tell one of the jokes I'd written specifically for the tour. Someone pitched a video package that included Woody Harrelson's brother Brett. One of the camera guys had gotten him walking up the Santa Monica stairs ON HIS HANDS. Harvey turned the conversation to the fact that Brett had been in the movie *The People vs. Larry Flynt* with Woody. He then told the room about how I believed that Larry Flynt, the now-deceased founder of *Hustler* magazine, was a true civil rights pioneer. The room was totally confused, but I wasn't.

On the tour, I would make a joke when we passed the

Hustler store on Sunset Boulevard. It was a joke to test the temperature of the crowd. I'd tell the bus that Larry Flynt was one of the most important people in civil rights history because reportedly he'd been shot by a gunman who was incensed about the interracial photos in *Hustler*. People on the tour, thinking this was the point of the story, would nod along in a very *I didn't know that* manner. I would then deliver the punch line, which was that Larry Flynt was a civil rights hero because he took a bullet so that I could fuck white women. I could guarantee that 95 percent of the time the bus erupted in laughter. The 5 percent of the time it didn't meant that the people were probably from Utah.

When Harvey took my tour, he lost it at that joke. And the first thing he did during my first show on TMZ was find a way for me to tell it. I remember knowing exactly what he was getting at when he said, "Van has an idea why Larry Flynt is actually a civil rights pioneer." Everyone turned to me. There was legit no sound. The only thing I could hear was my heart pounding in my neck. I almost got dizzy from the moment. But I pushed through it. As I set the joke up, the room still remained graveyard-quiet. But when I hit the punch line, they ERUPTED in laughter. I was now part of the group.

It didn't take long for me to realize that there was a culture problem at TMZ. I'd never really watched the show or visited the website before working there, so I didn't know much about the operation. I thought that it was a celebrity news and entertainment show similar to *Extra* or *Access Hollywood*.

After a while, I began to see the organization for what it really was. I was working for the renegades of celebrity news. TMZ sought to rewrite the Hollywood rules on how celebrities were covered—and they weren't going to apologize for this, either. On the contrary, it seemed like they wanted to piss off the industry. Everything from the headlines to the pictures they chose for the website was done to foster a belief in the inherent "otherness" of the celebrity experience. You never feel more human than when you're looking at animals in a zoo—and TMZ provided a zoo animal experience for the reader and the watcher. The animals were the celebrities, and othering them made you feel one with the brand.

That oneness between brand and consumer is also why it's impossible to beat TMZ in breaking videos. I know that people believe there's some sort of journalistic prestidigitation that goes on for TMZ to get all the huge videos they get, but there isn't. By and large, *they* don't get those videos; *you* do. Someone either takes the video on their camera phone or has access to it in some other way, and then they contact TMZ via the tip line. The tip line makes EVERYONE TMZ.

If you caught a lion out in the wild, you'd take it to a zoo. If you catch a celebrity out in the wild, you take it to TMZ.

I had been there about six months when I happened upon a video package featuring Wiz Khalifa. What was interesting to me was that under the footage there was text on the bottom of the screen that read LIL' BOW WOW. I'm not sure who confused the five-foot-seven Bow Wow with the six-foot-five Wiz Khalifa, but I'm sure it wasn't done to further a white-supremacist narrative. And the mistake reinforced my worth at TMZ; they needed someone to help them tell the difference between Bow Wow and Wiz, and they obviously didn't have that person. This was despite the fact that an amazing and talented Black woman named Nina Parker was working there, and no one knows more about pop culture and Black culture than she does. Still, that's the story I told myself: They needed me to be Black.

Being Black at TMZ was incredibly nerve-racking and made me feel very anxious at times. When they ran afoul of the Black community, because I was the Black guy, I'd take heat for it.

I remember when they did a video called "How to Shoot Black People." The piece was a gag on how our camera guys always got the lighting wrong whenever they'd spot Black celebrities on the street. Apparently, we had a bunch of funny clips of Black celebrities who were filmed so terribly that we couldn't tell who they were. At face value, this piece was fucked-up for many reasons. The whole gist of it was othering and lampooning our Black skin, and passively stating that it was a chore to film us. It was the whole American pie in one bad joke. We're extra, we're different, and you have to make a special effort to let us in. It was divisive for no reason.

To make matters worse, this segment aired in the aftermath of the Trayvon Martin killing. The call I got from a very prominent Black celebrity in response to that segment made me feel ashamed and angry. He'd gotten my number from a friend and, rightly so, he lit my ass up and said, "What's the purpose of you even being there if the bullshit is still going on?"

There was absolutely nothing that I could say in that moment, so I just shut the fuck up and let him continue.

"When I see you on there," he growled at me, "you look like you hold it down, but now I'm scratching my head, like how does something like this get on TV with you there?"

I took his verbal ass-whipping for about twenty minutes, because he was someone I'd watched since I was a kid and respected. What he didn't know is that I wasn't even in the office the day it happened.

That didn't matter, though, because whatever TMZ did, I had to answer for it. Rapper gets arrested with 150 guns in his tour bus? Van says he was targeted by police. Actor gets a DUI driving 150 miles an hour through a school zone? Van says they were in a hurry to pick up the kids and got carried away. I wasn't a person anymore; I became an avatar for my community.

The response I got from that video changed me fundamentally. I no longer felt I had the ability to be objective about Black celebrities. By the time TMZ had shifted, and a large portion of the website was now reporting on Black celebrities, the coverage was very often bereft of any type of social nuance. I felt I had no choice but to lose my nuance as well. I did this partly out of a desire to defend my community and partly out of a desire to defend myself. I'd never in life, EVER, been halfway considered an Uncle Tom, or a coon, or any of those disparaging words used to describe Black voices that the community deems off code. Now it was happening every week. I fought it tooth and nail.

Sometimes I fought it honestly, offering what I felt was genuine insight into things I felt TMZ was missing. Other times I fought blindly, proudly displaying a cultural cognitive dissonance. I'd carved out a real reputation that I was the guy who'd nail you if you came at the culture the wrong way. I'd also made enough salient points for people to know I knew what I was talking about. And my influence was growing. I became a producer, which meant I would sit with Harvey at his desk, write stories, or change headlines or language in posts when there were questions about how it would read.

I had the best of both worlds. A large part of the audience saw me as a voice of reason in a chaotic, hectic, and insensitive organization. Others saw me as the wisecracking know-it-all Black guy. Things were actually pretty good midway through my tenure there.

Then came Donald Trump.

When Trump first decided to run for president, I imagined, like many people, that his run would be good for his personal brand, and maybe even funny to watch. Despite all the birther nonsense he'd started by challenging Obama's American citizenship and having spats about that bullshit with liberal celebrities like Rosie O'Donnell and Whoopi Goldberg on *The View*, I didn't have very much of an opinion about Trump. He was a "billionaire" who was the host of *The Apprentice*. In my mind, there was no way his presidential run could ever lead to an honest win. Then two things happened: First, Trump became, almost overnight, a viable candidate for president, and second, TMZ got close with the Trump campaign. Harvey and Trump had known each other for a while, so no one was really surprised when Harvey joked about how frequently Trump called. However, many of us became alarmed when it seemed like

TMZ became a full-fledged propaganda machine. It was so obvious that the *Daily Beast* ran an article about it in 2018, accusing TMZ of going full MAGA.

I didn't read the article at the time, because I didn't need to. The results of our cozy relationship with Trump were evident all over the newsroom. Morale was lowering as the young, typically liberal staff reacted to being the new Fox News. Almost no one supported Trump, but Harvey seemed undeterred.

I'd been there just long enough to think that I mattered. Harvey had been there for me when I'd had anxiety issues and during times that my father was sick, and he'd helped develop me into what I became on the show. He was a charitable, decent guy who looked out for so many people, yet here I was, asking him and white America not to help an unabashed white supremacist get in the Oval Office, and I was ignored.

It didn't take Harvey long to turn against Trump after he was elected, but I never let it go. I couldn't. My relationship with Harvey deteriorated pretty rapidly after that. We were having ridiculously heated arguments during the shows. Although I don't know who Harvey voted for in the end, to me, the people who voted for Trump and then regretted it were the worst of all. They were the ones who'd refused to listen to reason. And they'd made him leader of the FREE FUCKING WORLD. How about you just listen to Black, Brown, and LGBTQ Americans when we tell you what's trying to hurt us? How about you turn the volume down on your privilege and turn it up on your compassion?

Still, I worked for TMZ until 2019, when I was fired after an altercation with a coworker. This was one of the most bizarre occurrences in my life. Harvey wasn't in the office. During the daily morning production meeting with the editors, there was a story about Ellen DeGeneres being friends with George W. Bush. I think that it is awesome that people like her and Michelle Obama have developed warm and friendly relationships with W. (Seriously, I mean that.) They don't have to feel the way I feel. I'm from South Louisiana. I have a problem with war criminals who leave Americans to drown in filthy water during the hottest month of the year. I have a problem with flyover photo ops while Louisianans drown. I'm not good with W, and I never will be.

During the morning meeting, I said just that, and I even got a little emotional, which I often do when talking about Hurricane Katrina. When it came time to do *TMZ Live*— which is a midday news roundup of all the stories of the day taped live—I specifically said I didn't want to discuss the Ellen connection with Bush. I said it over and over again.

My coworker Mike Babcock, who is very conservative but happens to be one of my favorite people on earth, got into it. It was very heated. On-screen, I played it off rather well. But during the commercial break, I went to tell Mike how I felt about the exchange. As I came up behind him, I put my hands on his shoulder. We argued, and as I was walking away, one of the executive producers of the show, told me that I should go home. It would be the last time I'd ever set foot inside of TMZ.

I was told the body contact with Mike was inappropriate and they had no choice but to let me go. I really couldn't have cared less. I had about six weeks left on my contract and had already told them I was out the door.

At first when I was fired, no one outside of TMZ knew. I wanted to think that everything was fine and the whole ordeal was behind me. In fact, that prior Saturday, my old coworkers—including Mike—had gotten together and thrown me a proper going-away party. It was an amazing goodbye to my time at TMZ.

Then one day, I got a call from a guy with Page Six of the *New York Post*. He told me they were preparing to run a story about my dismissal and wanted to know if I had any comment.

"No comment," I said. Then I proceeded to freak the fuck out.

I was petrified—petrified—because what did this mean now? Did this mean that nine years of me being who I am was now washed away? Did this mean that now I was angry, I was untouchable, there were going to be people who didn't want to work with me? I had been a peacemaker. I'd been someone who'd never been in any trouble. I'd been somebody who'd always tried to use the gifts that God has given me to bring people together and get them on the same side of things while telling the truth in a very plain way. Was all of that now gone?

I had to go see a cardiologist. I was walking around, and my heart was beating funny. I was smiling at my girl, but I felt completely unhealthy. I wasn't sleeping. I had to start taking beta blockers. I was gorging myself with junk food. I was scared.

In the end, the Page Six story turned out to be mild. The good news is, I had job offers for other TV shows and on-air opportunities from all over. And I had support from many people I respected in the Black community.

Second to the Kanye confrontation, being fired was the biggest moment of my career. A lot of people were fed up with TMZ's bullshit by this time.

The very next day, I was alerted to the fact that TMZ was going to leak a story to Page Six that showed my hands around Mike's throat (which they never were) and explaining that the reason why I was fired was because I got physical. Every single soul in that building knows I'd never do anything to hurt Mike Babcock. He was, and is, my friend and a good man, despite his fucked-up politics.

It was disingenuous and, in my opinion, an intellectual lie. It was also something else. Exactly what I deserved. I'm a spiritual man, and I don't believe God wanted me to leave TMZ without experiencing what being on the other side of a headline felt like. I'd earned this moment. A moment to understand that every headline is an actual human being, and not just a hot topic.

After TMZ came back with the second Page Six story, I felt like I'd thrown my entire career away. All the insecurity about not having a job, all the questions about what I would do next, started to haunt me. Would people want to work with me after this? I was a man who had never been arrested or violent, but I had still ended up playing into the stereotype of the dangerous, unhinged Black savage.

How could I have been so stupid? I thought over and over again. I had some of the worst anxiety I'd ever had in my life. People began talking bad about what happened to me in YouTube reaction videos, on podcasts, and on talk shows. It's a weird feeling trying to combat a narrative about yourself that you know isn't true. I thought about all the times I'd talked about people and their celebrity exploits without knowing them or the actual dynamics of the situation.

I promised myself that I'd never do that again. I'd never again be a part of an exploitative culture.

My time at TMZ was a part of my life that I'll never forget. I learned a lot and accomplished a ton. I both regret nothing and miss nothing. But I'm happy to have achieved something so many Americans don't have the opportunity to achieve—which is to actually enjoy what you do.

10

399 Yards of Deception

On December 22, 2003, the Green Bay Packers played the Oakland Raiders on *Monday Night Football*. The game itself was pretty inconsequential as far as NFL games go. Neither team had any real Super Bowl aspirations. There were no huge records that were going to be broken, and no football-related story lines to speak of. The game itself ended up being a stinker as well. The Raiders were enduring a miserable season and got walloped, 41–7, in the type of game that makes people complain about Monday night matchups—except no one was complaining about this game. The entire sports world was amazed. It became arguably the most legendary and memorable Monday night rout in the history of the NFL. The reason people talked about, and still talk about, that game is simple: grief.

Brett Favre, the quarterback of the Packers and an all-time NFL great, was playing this game not just as his team leader, but as a grieving son. His father, Irvin Favre, had died the night before of a sudden heart attack while driving in Brett's home state of Mississippi. Within hours, Favre had addressed his teammates, letting them know about the situation and telling them that he would be playing the next night against the Raiders.

He played and was brilliant. He threw for 399 yards and four touchdowns. Of those 399 yards, 311 of them came during the first half, which saw Favre completely overwhelm the Raiders with his right-armed brilliance. The game instantly became the stuff of legend. Favre was hailed as a hero for showing up to work and being amazing at a time when no one would have begrudged him for going into a hole somewhere to hide and cry. The game was legendary not because the Packers beat the Raiders, but because Brett Favre beat grief.

I kept it in my mind how brave Brett Favre was, and how

everyone remembered him for rising to the occasion and showing up for the people in his life despite a devastating loss. I kept saying it to myself: *Three hundred ninety-nine yards. Three hundred ninety-nine yards. Excellence in the face of trauma. Show up. Everyone needs you. Don't let them down.*

One day in July 2021, while I was writing this book, I got a call at six in the morning. *Too early to answer,* I thought. But then I heard Khalika's phone ring, too. Whoever it was had reached out to me and didn't get me, so they reached out to her. She was completely knocked out. When I looked at my phone to see who had called, it was my sister. As soon as I saw her name as the caller, I knew my father was dead.

My father had congestive heart failure for around twenty years. A hospital stay would have been no reason for my sister's frantic back-to-back calls. We'd done this over and over again, and the common denominator was that I'd assumed that he would always be around for a call later on. This time, my brain and my heart were doing a delicate dance with each other. They both knew what was going on, but I still had to pick up the phone and get the confirmation.

I called her back, and her voice confirmed the story: "Daddy died. He's gone." I didn't stay on the phone too much longer after that. I turned to Khalika and told her, and then my body started doing whatever it wanted to.

I couldn't catch my breath. I couldn't think. I couldn't

hear, and it felt like I couldn't see. My brain wasn't registering the things my eyes met. I looked at the TV, and my brain said, *Your father died.* I looked at my dog, and my brain said, *Your father died.* I sat on the floor for an hour, then got up and went and lay in my hammock, and eventually fell asleep. When I woke up, my friends were around me, gluing me together every second I threatened to break.

The next day, I flew back to Louisiana and began the process of laying my father to rest. I had to drive to his hometown of Maringouin and pick out the box he was going to rest in. While driving on the I-10 freeway, across the Mississippi River bridge, I thought about Brett Favre's legendary performance, and I couldn't understand how he did it. Every single aspect of this was excruciating for me, and I wanted to quit. I wanted to write a check to someone and have all of it taken care of while I sat in my sorrow somewhere. Only I couldn't. I'd heard from a half dozen people about how I was "the man of the family now" and how I needed to show up. So here I was, showing up.

Two of my best friends were making the ride with me, and while they talked to me about old times, I kept thinking about Brett, a man who didn't hesitate when it was time to step up for his teammates. Not only did he step up, but he had one of the greatest games of a Hall of Fame career.

Now it was my time. Everyone was watching me, and now I had to throw some touchdowns.

We got to the funeral home, and it looked just like you'd expect it to: drab, low-lit, and dour. There was a spirit of death inside the place, which you'd expect because they're in the death business. We moved into the office and began to talk about how Dad would be laid out, which casket to choose, what to say in his obituary, who to invite, and which priest would do the Catholic Mass. The conversation surrounding the death of the man who literally created me was being had very cavalierly. I lasted about twenty minutes, then I broke.

I felt my body getting ready to crack, so I ran out of the funeral home and into the South Louisiana afternoon. The air was moist and humid, a contrast from the cold and sterile environment I'd just been in. I looked out over a field and just stood there in it—grief. There was no rewind. No fast-forward. In order to meet this moment, I would have to greet this moment. A thought popped into my mind as I stood there:

Man, fuck that football game.

I had looked at what Brett Favre had done as overcoming grief, as beating it with his right arm. I thought that's what I had to do. But when it came time for me to face the Raiders, I ran.

I went back into the room, but I legit counted the seconds until it was time to leave. I checked out totally and just went blank and numb. I wasn't engaged and alert, like Brett had to be. Sharp and excellent, like he was that Monday night in Oakland. I was frail and small, and everyone saw it. For about a minute, I felt like a weakling. Then I remembered something: My father had died.

There's no playbook for that. There's no *way* to handle that. There's nothing I *had* to do. Nothing *needed* to happen. Sure, he had to get buried. He had to have his cowboy hat when he died. He needed his boots and his suit. Those things had to happen, but *I* didn't have to do them. If I wanted to roll up into a ball and cry, I'd earned that right from being his son for forty-one years. I didn't have any orders to follow, just feelings, and the best way to honor my father was to follow them.

The fact that Brett Favre's game is so legendary speaks to who we want to be as humans. We want to believe that by sheer will we can transcend the most devastating things that happen to us. We want to believe that at our worst moments we can produce our best selves. We need to believe that because we know that our worst moments will never stop happening. Being human is the grief Olympics, and you get medals not for winning, but for how well you lose.

So I set out on a new journey. Not to beat grief, but to

grieve well. Maybe that's what Brett was doing after all. Maybe football, something he'd shared an immense love for with his father, was Brett's way of saying goodbye. Maybe throwing for all those yards wasn't him defying grief; maybe it was him surrendering to it. For me, surrendering to my grief meant making peace with some things. This was insanely difficult.

Even at my age, there are so many firsts left in my life. Now every first for me is something my father will never see. My children will never know my father. He'll never have a cameo in a movie I produce. He'll never come to Christmas at my home. He'll never even see me own my own home. There's an entire piece of me that he won't know—which is weird, because he was one of the only human beings in the world who could say he'd been around for every piece of me.

I mourn my father. I mourn the man he was and the example he set. I mourn the rough way he communicated with people, including me. I mourn the five-thousand-megawatt smile he had. Hell, I even mourn the fearmongering, uncompromising dickhead he often was. But more than any of that, I miss what we hadn't done yet. I miss vacations we never took. Baseball games we never went to. Meals we never ate together. That's what grief is. It's saying goodbye to promises you never knew you wanted to make. I've been doing that ever since that day at the funeral home.

People from everywhere told me that I wouldn't go a day without thinking about him, and for now they're right. I recently got booked to do a gig in Japan, and the first thought I had was that my father never saw Japan. Make no mistake about it, my father had zero interest in seeing Japan; the very mention of sitting on a plane that long would've angered him to no end. But now, he'll never go. He can't change his mind. That whole stream of thoughts happened in about thirty seconds. It was like an emotional reflex. One that will probably be around for a little while. One that I have to make my peace with.

I talk to my father now more than I ever did when he was alive. That's a morbid and weird thing to think, and a harder one to type. As much as I revered my dad, he was hard for me to communicate with. I felt inadequate at the mere mention of him. He represented a type of manhood that I never felt like I could represent, even if I wanted to. For most of my life, it was as if we spoke two different languages, and neither one of us wanted to take classes in the way the other guy talked. After a while, we stopped attempting the translation. There was no beef per se; there just wasn't as much warmth as I think either one of us would've wanted.

In the place of the warmth, there was silence, which is normally what people use as a placeholder when there's no warmth. He was calling a lot in the months before he passed away, and we had some good conversations. Still, most of the time when he'd call, I'd find a reason to either cut the convo short or send the call to voicemail. Now it's different. I talk to him constantly.

I took a bone-handled knife that he owned with me from Louisiana. My dad had this thing he used to do with the knife. He'd spin it on his palm, then catch it and flick it out at the same time. This was dangerous. The knife was sharp. But, man, he'd nail it every time. Of course, now that I own the knife, I've tried to do the same thing. I made a ritual out of it. I looked in the mirror and spun the knife, trying to wield it like the first bearer of my name. After about three times of failing, I asked for help: "Jesus, Dad, how do you do this shit?" I caught myself after I did that, looked in the mirror, and cried a little. That's also grief. An unanswered question between father and son.

Now when I talk to my father, I say things to him that I never had the balls to say when he was alive. Even though there's nothing coming back, the words are more than sounds—and they are just as difficult to say. I realize that as much as I miss my father now, the truth is that I've missed him for years. I've missed him since I was about fifteen years old. I tell him I wish things would've been different with us. I tell him I'll remember and honor him until they remember and honor me. More than anything, though, every single day, I tell my father I love him.

When I started writing this chapter I was determined to tell everyone what I've learned about grief. If I'm being honest, I haven't learned that much about grieving. I have, however, learned about me. I've learned that I'm not the kind of guy who throws for 399 yards the day after his father passes away. I'm the guy who runs crying out of the funeral home after someone asks what kind of casket to put his dad in.

Grieving this hard has taught me what I can handle and what I owe myself. I owe myself space. Space to play football or not play football. Space to talk to Dad or be silent. Space to handle everything or handle nothing. I can't do anything more than that, and I can't do anything less. There's still a tough road ahead of holidays, birthdays, weddings—all without Van Terry Lathan Sr. That's hard. That's final.

I can't run from that, and I shouldn't run toward it, either. I'll just walk. And if you see me crying or talking to my father, gimme some space.

11

Winner, Winner, Still a Sinner

I'm in a room full of people who are there because of me. Actually, they are there because of *us*. When I say *us*, I am referring to one of the most powerful collection of *us*es anyone could ever put together. We made something that broke through and got to people—in the middle of a pandemic, no less—so much so that this party is an Oscar party. My nerves are through the roof.

Until you've done it, you have no idea what waiting to

find out if you're a part of history feels like. I'll try to make it make sense with a sex analogy. Imagine your biggest celebrity crush told everyone that they wanted to have hot, passionate sex with you. This would be the type of lovemaking that you and everyone else would remember forever. You are prepared for it to happen on this one particular night, and everybody knows the exact time and place. Some are even watching. You dress up for the occasion, get a fancy ride over, and take your seat in one of the most lush and elegant rooms in the world. You wait, and then your crush walks out and tells you, "Not tonight." You ask when, and they say, "Maybe in the future, maybe never. But, hey, at least I considered you." You do what everyone should do when denied sex: You get up to leave and act like a grown-up, maybe even congratulate those who are having it. You put on your best smile. But when it's just you, by yourself, the thought going through your mind is that you wanted to fuck. You didn't come all that way to not get the experience and see it through. Sure, everyone knows that the hottest person in the world had some desire for you, but it means nothing compared to what the experience would've been like. Part of you would wish that you'd never even gotten that close at all.

That's exactly how I was feeling the night of the Oscars. A film that I executive-produced, *Two Distant Strangers*, was nominated for best live action short film at the Ninety-Third Academy Awards. The film was written by Travon Free and directed by Travon and Martin Desmond Roe, and the two of them came together to create a stunningly poignant and powerful piece of work. These two guys are insanely talented, and they were backed up by my partners at Six Feet Over Productions, the incredible production company Dirty Robber, and the creative genius of Jesse Williams and Lawrence Bender.

The movie went from concept to production to product to Oscar contender in a dizzying amount of time. We were all equal parts exhausted and awed with the process by the time Oscar night came around. For me, it was a weird time. I'd gained weight over the past months as I battled intense depression. I didn't look my best for the biggest moment in my creative life, and I didn't feel my best, either. I was going through the emotional and physical exhaustion that only stress can deliver, and I could no longer do an adequate job of hiding it. My prescription for it was to shut myself off from everybody, spending all day in the hammock or walking outside until my feet blistered. I'd begun to cut myself off from Khalika, my dog, and anything I didn't have to do.

For the entire time we were making this push for the movie to get recognized, I was struggling to hold on to any source of light in my life. This enormous accomplishment was right around the corner, and I couldn't grasp the meaning of it. It felt like it was happening to someone else. I didn't recognize me, so I couldn't connect the feeling of all this to my life experience. It was really the most punishing irony ever. Winning an Oscar was something I'd dreamed about my entire life. But for most of the campaign, I could only think of one thing: I didn't feel well, and I didn't know when I would again.

The night of the party was slightly different, though. I still had a pandemic-depression fog over me, but the energy of everyone pushed me forward. Sure, I was portly, pudgy, and sad, but everyone kept reminding me of how insane an occurrence this was. We had a small party at Hyde Sunset, which was supposed to be for production and a few friends but ended up being for whoever we loved who was vaccinated.

It was at the party that I realized how much I missed people. I'd been in the habit of incubating my problems. A problem would develop, I'd recognize it had developed, and I'd check on it every single day. At the party, I couldn't do this. People stopped me from incubating. They had their own jokes, their own outfits, and their own stories. I had to listen, I had to laugh, and I had to disagree. The atmosphere inside Hyde made me stop incubating, and the moment I did, I felt something else: nervousness.

I remember sitting down at a table, one that had a placard with my name on it (shout-out to my partner Nic Maye for getting it all done), and hearing Khalika say to me, "You're going to win an Oscar tonight! How does that feel?"

It had been a long time since my body felt nerves. My body was addicted to real anxiety at this point. Weirdly enough, the nerves settled me in. It was a familiar feeling, almost a relic of a time when there were things to be excited about. I was around people who loved me, respected me, and were rooting for me. I felt weirdly at ease.

Then the Oscars started.

This wasn't your traditional Oscars watch party. Most Oscars watch parties are about witnessing the spectacle of the awards themselves and debating the winners and losers. Our party was going to be either a coronation or condolences, so the tenor of the evening was different. We basically didn't give a fuck who won or lost anything else outside of Chadwick Boseman for best actor for *Ma Rainey's Black Bottom*.

The music was loud, people were talking, and there was a DJ to clue us in to when the best short film category was coming on.

Then the DJ said, "EVERYBODY LOOK AT YOUR SCREENS. LET'S GOOOOO!"

The music piped down, and it was finally time to actually

watch the Oscars. The presenter of the category was Riz Ahmed, the spectacular actor who was nominated for his amazing turn in *Sound of Metal*. He started reading the names of the films. The moment was huge. I imagine it's like watching your kid sing a solo in a choir. You're happy for everyone, but you came to see how one kid would do, and it's time now.

Riz wasted no time when he was done with the list of nominees. He said, "AND THE OSCAR GOES TO . . . *TWO DISTANT STRANGERS!*"

I threw my hat at the screen. The room erupted in tears and hugs. COVID and depression no longer exist. Only joy. We did it.

When I was sixteen, I told a teacher I'd win an Oscar someday. This is when I first realized that teachers have the hardest job in the world. My history teacher, Mrs. Smith, was tough with me. I was long on talent, full of dreams, but rudderless. Mrs. Smith said, "Do you even know what that means?"

In my mind, the Oscars were the Super Bowl of movies, where you go to win a filmmaking championship. That's not wrong per se, but it doesn't begin to describe what it takes to get there. At that age, I had no clue the sacrifice and focus it took to be a Super Bowl champion, and I certainly didn't know what it took to get a movie green-lit, paid for, produced, and distributed. My answer to Mrs. Smith was more flippant and smart-ass than anything. I looked at her and I said, "Do *you* know what that means, and if you do, why are you teaching?"

As I took my pink slip to the office, I remember realizing that Mrs. Smith knew me well, and she knew that the surest way to get me to learn about something was to insinuate that I didn't know what I was talking about. From that day on, I was obsessed with the Academy Awards. I watched every show every year, read up on the winners, the losers, and the snubs, and saw all the movies. I looked at the Academy Awards as something separate from filmmaking itself, and the ultimate validation of a childhood spent staring into story. Everyone knew what I wanted to do, and everyone knew I wouldn't be happy doing much of anything else. But as I got older, it became obvious that Mrs. Smith really knew what the fuck she was talking about: I had no idea how to get to where I wanted to be in life.

As the years passed, I was settling into my existence in Baton Rouge and I wasn't thinking about the Oscars much anymore. But that all changed when Hurricane Katrina hit Louisiana, which prompted me to relocate to Los Angeles. Within three years of living in LA, I had moved to Franklin and La Brea in Hollywood, literally around the corner from the Dolby Theatre, where the Academy Awards are held.

Every year, the ceremony would impact my life. It's a massive undertaking. Streets are shut down, and security is omnipresent—there are LAPD tanks on the streets. I'd always known getting an Academy Award was a big deal. I'd been telling everyone I was going to get one since I was sixteen years old. But it took me being right around the corner from the Oscars to realize just how far away from them I was.

Being in LA made me appreciate more what all this stuff is about. Getting validation from places like the Academy starts to mean less when you understand just how hard it is to get your ideas out. As a creative in this town, you start to care less about how what you make is received, and more about just the fucking opportunity to make it. Especially if you're Black, Asian, Latino, or a woman, and so on. Living that close to the theater actually made me come to resent the Academy Awards. I watched the show less and less.

Working at TMZ made me feel a million miles away from being who I wanted to be, even though I kept hope alive that one day I would make movies. I remember a specific time at TMZ when we were covering an actor in an Oscar campaign. They'd done something stupid, and their Academy Award win was in jeopardy. One of my coworkers in the office said, "Well, that's something that no one in this room will ever have to worry about, winning an Oscar."

Everyone laughed. I immediately launched into a rebuttal: "NO, NO, NO, that's something YOU will never have to worry about. DON'T SPEAK FOR ME." My reaction may seem like supreme confidence, but it really wasn't. It was fear that my coworker was right, fear that I'd packed it up. I wanted to believe, like most people do, that one day I would be who I'd said I was going to be when I was sixteen.

The night of the Oscars was a champagne-filled blur. Too many text messages to count and too many emails to read. This went on for weeks. I was acknowledged by my college. There were articles written about me in Baton Rouge newspapers, segments done about me on the news. The mayor of Baton Rouge, Sharon Weston Broome, interviewed me. This was as close to being who I'd said I was going to be as I can remember. Everyone back home was talking about me; everyone in LA was talking about us, the guys who'd made a movie during a pandemic and won an Oscar for it.

For weeks after, people would ask me the same question about the win: HOW DO YOU FEEL? It's a sensible question when you've just accomplished something remarkable. I'd hear it from everyone—my mother, my sister, former coworkers, even people on the street. The more people would ask me how I felt, the more I'd give the same answer. I'd smile real big, look them in the eye, and say, "Man, it's indescribable." I wasn't lying. It was an indescribable feeling that I had regarding the win, without a doubt. Exactly what was indescribable about it was more vexing to me. It wasn't that I couldn't describe the elation that I felt—it was that I couldn't describe the emptiness.

As soon as Oscar night ended and the nervousness subsided, reality had come back. We were still in a pandemic, and I was still depressed. I still slept until eleven and took four different prescription drugs to function through a day. Part of me had thought that if we won, I could ride that victory out of the fog. That didn't happen at all, and instead there was now the birth of a fear: the fear that no matter what happened to me in my life, I'd always be in crisis. I was afraid that whatever glitch in my spirit caused me to be anxious would break through anything that might happen to me.

As I write this part of my book, my dog—Boseman—is right next to me. He's an amazing companion. We've turned a corner in our relationship, because he's learned how to get up onto the bed and sleep right beside me. Boseman's a Bernedoodle, and he's about ninety-five pounds. When he lies next to me and puts his head on the pillow, it's almost like he's a human being. Me and the dog feel like best friends. Even still, it's hard for me to enjoy being with him and hanging out with him, because my mind keeps reminding me that there's a day when I'll have to say goodbye. With every lick and cuddle, I anticipate an unknown but certain pain, and it robs me of the moment I'm in with my best boy.

I was expecting to not feel this way with the Academy Award. I was expecting the validation from it to be something I could sink my teeth into. I thought that, for once, I'd be happy and content with the reality of life. When that didn't happen for me, my anxiety ramped up to a million percent. What would it take for me to be able to exhale?

My dad called me in late April, a couple days after the Oscar win. He wanted to know what an Academy Award was and why people kept bothering him about it. He asked me to reach out to everyone in the family and tell them to stop bothering him about some damn award he'd never even heard of. My father couldn't understand why people were calling *him* about an award *I'd* won. "I ain't won no goddamn award," he said. "Why you calling my phone?" I've never had a funnier conversation. People talk shit about the South, and I get that some of it is warranted. But the call with my father reminded me why I wouldn't want to be from any other region of any other place in the world. Southerners have the politest way of either reminding you that you aren't shit, or making you think you're the most important person in the world.

During this conversation with my father, I remembered something that I already knew, and that is the clear and present rule of NEC. NEC is a rule, a mantra, and a slogan all in one. It's something I started saying in high school but abandoned for some reason as I confronted adulthood. I used to scribble it everywhere. If you picked up a journal, a basketball, a football, a backpack, anything that belonged to me, you'd see it.

The blissful beauty of NEC dawned on me during an argument my uncles were having after Evander Holyfield beat the dog shit out of Mike Tyson back in the late '90s. We'd called everyone over to the house to watch the fight, and it wasn't going the way people wanted it to. My house was a Tyson house, and from the minute the fight started it was obvious Holyfield didn't come to play any games. As the fight progressed, Mike started to get his ass tended to more and more, and my uncles became rowdy. One of them started to argue that Tyson had always been over-rated and that it was blasphemy for anyone to have ever compared him to Muhammad Ali. As the Coors Light flowed more readily through their veins and the fight got more out of hand in Holyfield's favor, they got louder and louder, to the point where I had to intervene. It was right then and there that NEC was created. Me, a seventeen-year-old nephew, yelled at his uncles, "NOT EVERYONE CARES."

I'd use this phrase for years after to free me of the notion that everything was about me, that all of my ups and downs seismically shifted everything for everyone else. I'd, of course, also use it to remind other people that I didn't really care about their shit sometimes. I probably overused it to that effect, honestly, but still it was a good mantra to keep me focused on what was in front of me.

As I got older, it was harder to not care about things, no matter how small they were. It seemed every year raised the stakes on what I was supposed to care about, and how much. Add social media to that, and now it's insanely difficult to let anything slide. People tell you that if you don't care about certain things, you're a bad person, and up for cancellation. But the reality is, no matter what it is we're talking about, *not everyone cares.*

The conversation with my dad reminded me of that. I thought I'd feel different if we won, that I'd be different if we won—and then we did, and nothing really changed. My father, the man who gave me his whole life so that I could do what I was doing, didn't even care that I'd won. As much as that should've bothered me, it didn't. It freed me from thinking that any one thing is supposed to change how I'm feeling. That idea makes it seem like there's some sort of shortcut or cheat code to understanding what my life is about, and there obviously isn't. Life isn't a sprint or a marathon; it's a recipe. Some things get sweeter as you get older, some things get saltier, but in order to season to taste you have to know yourself.

Of course, there could be other reasons why the Oscar win hasn't filled me up. I didn't get to go to the awards or stand on the stage. It was Travon Free and Martin Desmond Roe's moment, and as the leading creatives on the film they overly deserve the shine. So maybe me feeling not totally fulfilled from it means that I'm selfish enough to want a moment where everything is about me. Where everyone looks at me and says, *There he is—it's the genius Van Lathan, and he's everything he thought he ever was.*

In a moment like that, where I've created something that everyone loves and worships, maybe I'd feel like I know why I'm supposed to be here. Maybe that'd make everything make sense. I'd be there in front of everyone, in great shape and wearing a tux from a Black designer. Maybe I'm selfish enough as a person that I need everything to be about me. Maybe I'm so emotionally clogged that I'll never be enough to myself and I need the validation of others in a very specific way to make me feel good about myself. Maybe I should try to enjoy my dog while he's here. Maybe I should try to enjoy the fact that we reached the heights of our industry on sheer will, guile, and talent. Maybe I should understand that the gift of life is living it, and not what happens in it.

That last sentence sounds like some supersoul Sunday bullshit, but that doesn't mean it's not true. I keep telling myself that I'll be happier "when," and then when the *when* comes, I'm the same kid I was when I was sixteen. When I don't have to worry about money. When I live in Los Angeles. When I'm not lonely. All these whens and no wins—it's a frustrating cycle.

At forty-one, part of me feels like I'm still waiting for my life to begin. Like there's something that's going to happen that's going to ignite a feeling of oneness or serenity with the space I live in. When I was losing the weight, my church was the scale. I'd skip a meal or two, and my body would let me know. My stomach would growl, and my energy would be low. Then I'd pop on the scale, and it would talk to me. It'd say, *Look, you're doing the right thing. Your pain is actually progress. Keep going.*

I think that's what I'm looking for more than anything: a promise that my pain is progress. I want a life scale, something to let me know that I'm going the right way or doing the right thing. For some reason, I thought winning an Oscar would do that. It didn't.

Winning reminded me that I'm right to think that I can do anything I put my mind to. It reminded me that I've been blessed to know some of the most talented and hardworking people in the world. It reminded me that these people are worth knowing forever. It also reminded me that my life probably isn't going to be defined by who recognizes me. I could be wrong, but I don't think I'm going to ever look at a collection of awards or dollar signs and say, "Okay, I can die now." The question is: What would make me feel okay about making that statement? What am I here chasing if not Oscars? Is peace within myself achievable for me? I don't know, and I bet you don't, either.

In the greatest movie franchise of all time, *Star Wars*, the greatest teacher of all time, Yoda, says something while training a brash and impatient Luke Skywalker on Dagobah. He instructs Luke to lift his X-wing fighter plane out of a swamp pond using the Force.

Luke turns to Yoda and says, "All right, I'll give it a try."

Yoda immediately responds with a deadly barb, "Do. Or do not. There is no try."

Luke then fails to do so and says it's impossible. But Yoda proves it is possible by lifting the plane out of the pond pretty easily.

Luke says, "I don't believe it."

Yoda then says, "That is why you fail."

I love you, Yoda, but this is some bullshit. Yoda is almost a thousand years old. He's been Force-lifting planes and shit for hundreds of years. Luke is like twenty-two. Come on, Yoda, be better than that. The "There is no try" is utter nonsense. The try is all we have. Our whole lives, our entire existence is an exercise in try. If you take the try from us, we're left with a world that's just winners and losers. If that's the case, what do you say to a guy like me who won but still feels unfulfilled? Am I supposed to chase a bigger win? A more self-serving one? If there is no try, then how do winning or losing provide us with any lessons?

I don't have any answers, but if I was a betting man, I'd wager that life is about the lessons and not the results. When I sit and think about it, winning the Oscar wasn't about winning at all. It was about creating and connecting with amazing people. Feeling the rush of watching actors like Zaria, Joey Badass, and Andrew Howard perform up close. The whole thing was in the try, Yoda. The try is the trophy.

But still, I'd like to thank the Academy.

12

Can I Live?

Now that I'm in my forties, my age seems ancient and not nearly old enough at the same time. I rarely feel my age these days, which both amazes and scares me. The only times I'm reminded of how many years I have on me is when I talk to younger people. I'm constantly astounded at the blissful and exuberant wrongness of youth.

The older you get, the more you realize that living is a constant negotiation. You negotiate how much you want to sleep as compared with the quality and productivity of the next day. You negotiate how much you eat with the size of your jeans. You negotiate how hard you work with the amount of time you spend with your family. Getting older for me is just a reminder that there was a time when I didn't need to compromise. There was a time when I could do whatever I wanted and just thug it out in the aftermath. Youth gives you that power. It's rebellion. It's chaos. It's not knowing and not caring. It's the belief that you always have another chance to get it right, another day to fight, and another battle to win.

I do a podcast with a brilliant young man, Charles, where we talk about the latest in nerd culture. If you don't know what nerd culture is, it's basically anything that you got teased for liking in 1995, such as comic books, anime, and superhero movies. There's a portion of our podcast where me and Charles recap episodes of shows in thirty seconds. Or at least it started out as thirty seconds. I was so bad at doing the quick recap that we had to move it to forty seconds, which I still struggle with. One week, Charles had to do the recap, and he nailed it in twenty-eight seconds. He's an insanely good podcaster, so this didn't surprise me.

But the next week, I was getting ready to do the recap, and I had our producers put forty seconds on the clock.

Charles said, "You don't want to try it in under thirty, like I did last week?"

I was like, "No, it's not a competition."

He said, "Everything is a competition. Life is a competition."

I thought about that for a second—a split second—and replied with a statement that finally convinced me that my years on this earth have translated into at least a little wisdom.

I told Charles, "Life isn't a competition. Life is peace. The older you get, the more you'll understand that."

Crazy thing is that it wasn't until that moment that I actually understood it for myself. Peace is the answer to every question I've asked in my life. It's what we all are reaching for. We don't really know what happens when we're done on this earth.

Don't get me wrong—I have faith. But even using that word *faith*, I can't be sure of what that experience will look and feel like. Deep down, we know that this moment is all we can really be certain of. Every moment we waste in chaos is an eternal chance missed. We all know we have to spend some time in the chaos cycle. The question is, though: How much time?

This is what health means to me now. Mental health means mental peace. Physical health means physical peace. Financial health means financial peace. Spiritual health means spiritual peace. It's that simple.

I remember what it was like living life at 360 pounds. It

was a constant war with my body. My movement, my gut health, my sleep—everything was affected by the amount of weight I was carrying. I couldn't find a peaceful existence with myself at that size, but I still sought it. I knew moving was a struggle, so I stayed still. I knew being seen was stressful, so I stayed hidden. I knew food brought me comfort, so I comforted myself. I was trying to achieve a feeling of just being okay. But in truth, I didn't know what okay was. We spend a lot of our lives being wrong about what okay is. Finding okay takes work, experience, and experimentation.

In 2016, I was sitting at my desk at TMZ when I felt dizzy. I box, and there's something that happens when you get caught with a really good punch. You get a fleeting moment of dizziness, mixed with panic, mixed with a jolt of *Wake up!* It's basically your body saying, *We didn't like that. Don't do that again.* When you're in a fight, this feeling makes you focus, either on the man in front of you, or on the sound of your coach. Sometimes you can actually see boxers shake a shot off to get their bearings back.

Now imagine feeling that jolt while you're just sitting down, with no one in front of you pounding on your face. A jolt of dizziness and panic like you just caught a right hook. I decided to get up and walk it off. I got about fifteen feet before the dizziness hit me like a tidal wave, and I fell completely over.

I could see the faces of my coworkers change as I tumbled in almost slow motion. Some of their eyes bulged. Some of them began to laugh, thinking I was joking. Some of them screamed. I never lost consciousness, but I lay there for a second. I'd managed to fall into the viewing room, where producers were watching the feed of the show before it went out, and they rushed over to me.

Before I knew it, I was hooked up to an EKG and on my way to the hospital again. I got checked out, released, and sent home.

The dizziness would last for a month. I was out of work the entire time. No one could figure out what was wrong with me. I had a full workup: cardiac, neurological, internal. Everything checked out. I was in great shape and had just come off a vacation. This didn't make sense. I couldn't walk more than fifty steps without feeling intense fear. That's what my anxiety was like at that time in life. I was literally tiptoeing around LA, waiting for something terrible to happen. But with each medical doctor I spoke to, I had a clean bill of health.

The consensus from all my doctors was becoming that my issues may be due to anxiety. And one day, a neurologist I was seeing in Beverly Hills suggested that I give therapeutic yoga a try. Weirdly, there was some aversion on my part. Here I was, taking every drug they prescribed to me, with all the advertised side effects, but for some reason, trying therapeutic yoga was vexing to me. I put it off for weeks as I underwent further testing. This testing was all by my request. I had them test for everything from Parkinson's disease to ALS. Whatever I could google, I had them work me up for it.

Eventually, they sent the yoga practitioner into an exam room I was in. She looked exactly like most yogis look to me. She was small and lean, but not overly muscular. She was Indian and had a subtle accent.

She looked at me and said, "Such a strong soul. Why are you afraid of healing?"

I cried.

She looked at me and said, "Sit up straight."

I did.

She then said, "Lift your chin. Clear your chest of confusion."

I followed her instructions.

Then she said, "Breathe."

I said, "I am breathing."

She said, "No. Breathe on purpose."

As I began to breathe on purpose, a wave of calm entered my body. I felt, at least for a second, that the gravity in the room was secure.

We began to meet once a week for therapeutic yoga. Yoga

pushed me to understand my breath and my body in a way that I can't describe. We would breathe in different ways, some that were actually challenging to learn. The sessions lasted an hour, and in that time it was pure serenity.

Breathing on purpose made me feel like I was created on purpose. That's what my anxiety takes from me—my purpose. It makes me feel like I was created for fear, and not for anything else. I'd get into waves where every day was about how to cope. Yoga practice took me out of that loop, slowed the world down, and brought me back to baseline. After about three weeks of practice, I returned to work.

I'd love to tell you that I unlocked the secret of serenity and that my life was forever changed, but that isn't true. After I started feeling better, I had a decision to make. There was a supercompetitive basketball league that played its games in downtown LA on Thursday nights. But Thursday nights were the only time I had to do yoga. Of course I chose basketball, and I haven't been back to yoga since.

What I've learned about myself is that the biggest road-block to my peace is me. It's not the world around me. It's not my childhood or my genetics. It's the man in the mirror. Finding peace takes work. You have got to want it *bad*. Sometimes you'll have to add things to your life to find it. Sometimes you'll have to subtract things from your life to find it.

There's no better example of this than what happened during the pandemic in 2020 and 2021. The entire world was forced to push the PAUSE button on their distractions, and what happened? Did we all just chill and find parts of ourselves that we hadn't had time to seek out before? NO. We went fucking crazy.

Why is this? A lot of the chaos in our lives was gone. We had time to do whatever we wanted to do for a while, and no one could say anything. Endless time to delve into who and what we are. And what did we realize? Two things: One, fear is tough to beat. Having an invisible demon lurking around every corner means it's hard to relax. Fear is the number one enemy of peace, and we all came to realize this while we were putting our groceries in the dishwasher during COVID, just to be sure. Two—and this is the more daunting and somewhat sobering realization—many of us found we didn't know our purpose. When the chaos, hustle, and bustle were removed from our lives, a lot of us didn't know who we were. What if there's no deadline? What if there's no meeting? What if there's no party, no loud music, and no traffic? What happens then?

I found that a lot of the chaos I have in my life I'd placed there to distract me from having to deal with the fact that I didn't have any peace. Getting drunk does that, having random sex does that (that'll be another book), even playing my beloved basketball can do that. When I go out and hoop until I can't anymore, I don't pay attention to the fact that I'm not taking any time for myself or getting to know more about myself. But over the course of the pandemic, I learned—and I think we all learned—that taking time for yourself doesn't matter if you don't know what to do with yourself.

As a Black man in America, peace seems impossible to me sometimes. As a matter of fact, it's frowned upon in some places. Sometimes in our community, we believe that the more chaos you've conquered, the worthier a man you are. The more serene your upbringing was, the less worth you have. This is both an infuriating dynamic to live with and a totally understandable one. Black Americans have had maybe the least peaceful existence of any group in America. Every part of our experience has been violent. Because of that, sometimes we see the people who're the worthiest as the people who have the most scars.

The first time this hit home for me was with my friend Delvin. Delvin was a guy from my neighborhood who I'd known since middle school. We lost touch for the first couple years of high school because he went to a different school than me. However, when we both found ourselves in summer school after the tenth grade, we clicked back up.

Delvin used to pick me up in the morning and drop

me off in the evening, something my dad appreciated so much that he'd give Delvin cash whenever he saw him. My father carried a gigantic .357 Magnum, which Delvin saw whenever they'd interact. He'd tell everyone about it, saying, "Van daddy got that iron. Don't fuck with him."

One day when we got to school, Delvin said something about my sister's butt, and I punched him playfully. Only when I hit him in his upper hip area, I hurt my hand. There was something in his waistband. I was like, "What's that?" In the parking lot of Christian Life Academy, Delvin pulled a .380 pistol out of his waistband. "Yo daddy ain't the only one got iron," he said.

My father routinely paid the men who worked for him with cash, so he carried large sums of cash on him. The gun was a deterrent from anyone trying him. He was never robbed.

Delvin was different for me. I couldn't see a reason he'd be carrying a gun—TO SCHOOL. Sure, we lived in Gardere, a decently rough neighborhood in Baton Rouge, but it wasn't an *ABC Afterschool Special*. We weren't looking over our shoulders 24/7, waiting to be taken out by the streets. At least I wasn't.

That day at school, I thought about Delvin's sidearm. And when we left that day, I asked him about it. He told me there were definitely guys who wanted to kill him, and he couldn't let his guard down no matter where he was. Before I asked him why, I noticed something. The minute I'd asked him about the gun, he began to smile. As he drove, he was still smiling. He then told me something I'll never forget. He said I was cool as hell and fun to be around, but the only thing missing from my personality was that I hadn't "done any dirt."

Doing dirt, where I'm from, means doing illegal and sometimes violent shit. Delvin then tried to convince me that guys in the neighborhood, and even some girls, weren't really going to respect me unless they knew I was "'bout that action." It was then that I realized why Delvin was smiling. He was smiling because he enjoyed carrying the gun. And he enjoyed it not because he loved guns, but because he was proud he was dangerous enough to need it.

Where I grew up, it's not peace that makes you whole; it's danger. You protect what little serenity you have by convincing the entire world that you'll kill them if they try to take it. Delvin was telling me that I was too straightlaced for anyone to feel that I would hurt them. That meant they couldn't feel totally safe around me, which meant there were some friendships I just wouldn't have and some girls I just couldn't get with. My environment was teaching me that my peace was my enemy. Peace would only invite people to try me, according to guys like Delvin—so it was worthless.

Around four years after that, Delvin was murdered at the Texaco station in our neighborhood. I'm still not sure what actually happened, but I know it was a fight, a gun got pulled, and he lost his life. When I told my father, he couldn't believe it. He never saw it in Delvin. I wouldn't have either if not for that conversation in the car.

As Black men, we always say we don't want to be seen as dangerous, and a lot of us mean that. But are there some of us who feel like we're not sharp and ready for the horror of America if we're not on the defensive? Are we okay as Black men with the peace that comes with being loved and not feared?

For some of us, the fear has protected us for so long. We feel like we're the survivors of something that's not easy to survive—being Black in America—so we don't want to lose the edge that has protected us. And when war has defined you—war against poverty, war against violence, and war against racism—how do you let peace in? Can you let peace in?

My friend Geno and I came up with a mantra back in our early twenties after a string of our friends had died. We're talking murders back-to-back-to-back. Geno looked at me one day and said, "Man, I just want to live." I agreed. Losing so many people around us made me think that just existing was enough.

With more than forty years on me, I now know that's not enough. I have to have peace. It's the number one priority in my life. Not money, not fame. Peace. I work at it every day.

Finding peace at this point in my life means therapy, honesty, and realization. The realization is that it's okay for me to find peace and be peaceful. I don't owe America, the world, or white supremacy anything. My anger and frustration don't do anything to change those entities. Only love for myself, and love for the Black and human community, can make me whole.

It's not that I'll never be angry. It's that I won't ONLY be angry. It's not that I'll never be violent. It's that I won't ONLY be violent. It's not that I'll never be scared. It's that I won't ONLY be scared. For me, finding peace means not ruminating on what will go wrong, because something always will. If the last two years of my life—when I lost my job and my father, and we all lost our way—have taught me anything, it's that.

But long walks are still there. Therapy is still there. The love of an amazing and supportive partner is still there. Peace is still there, and that's what I seek.

I wonder about my younger Black brothers and contemplate if they know that not having an enemy is okay. If they know it's okay to be okay. I wonder how we find peace in a society where the trees were fertilized with the blood of our ancestors. I think about those ancestors and what they would've wanted for us. How their lives were made of forced struggle, overwhelming and superhuman sacrifice, and, of course, pain. I think they would have wanted us to make a better life for each other. But they would've also just wanted us to be. To peacefully exist in the land they built.

I refuse to give my peace to a country or a society that doesn't deserve it, but I absolutely will give it to myself and the people I love. That's worth it.